CW00371458

WOMEN AND HEALTH

WOMEN AND HEALTH
An Introduction To Issues

DEBORAH SALTMAN
School of Community Medicine, University of New South Wales

assisted by Sally Redman (chapters three, seven and eight)
and Sue Irvine (case studies)

HARCOURT BRACE JOVANOVICH, PUBLISHERS
Sydney   London   Orlando   San Diego   Toronto

This book is dedicated to my father Kurt Saltman, my sister Dr Maureen Waine and especially my mother, Bronia Saltman, who germinated these ideas but did not live to see them grow. I miss her warmth and spontaneity, she will always be the guiding light of my life.

Harcourt Brace Jovanovich Group (Australia) Pty Limited
30–52 Smidmore Street, Marrickville NSW 2204

Harcourt Brace Jovanovich Limited
24/28 Oval Road, London NW1 7DX

Harcourt Brace Jovanovich Inc.
1250 Sixth Avenue, San Diego, California 92101–4311

Copyright © 1991 by Harcourt Brace Jovanovich Group (Australia) Pty Limited

This publication is copyright. Except as expressly provided in the Copyright Act 1968, no part of this publication may be reproduced by any means (including electronic, mechanical, microcopying, photocopying, recording or otherwise) without prior written permission from the publisher.

Printed in Australia

National Library of Australia Cataloguing in Publication Data

Saltman, Deborah.

Women and health: an introduction to issues.

Includes index.
ISBN 0 7295 0285 6.

1. Women's health services. 2. Women — health and hygiene.

362.83

Contents

Introduction

The catch cry 'women's health' has suffered from much moral indignation and out-rage. Women's health is seen as gynocentric, hysteric, alienating, aggressive and, more commonly, elitist. The mere term leads to a knee jerk reaction: why not study class or race issues of health? Why not study men's health? And, indeed, these are not questions which can be answered easily. That is why we have chosen to write about 'women *and* health'. Under this banner we can explore the inter-relationships between women and both the formal and informal health care con-text in which they find themselves.

In order to strengthen women's relationship with health care in Australia, we must first identify the current status. This is not easy, perhaps that is why this is the first book of its kind to attempt what is almost an impossible task. First of all we must decide which set of topics should be addressed. However, as women are both the major consumers and providers of health care in this country, the provider/consumer nexus created the framework for the text of this book. In writ-ing about the inequities in health care for women we are not saying that health care has adverse effects only for women, or that the adverse effects apply to women equally. But nevertheless, some of the topics raised apply only to women — for ex-ample chapter 7, which discusses reproduction issues. Then again some chapters deal with different applications of health for men and women — for example chap-ter 3, which assesses women's health needs.

As there is a dearth of material in Australia addressing these issues, we have tried to tackle as many as possible. Some issues are covered in more depth, particularly when recent Australian data is available. For example in chapter five, Women as Providers and Consumers of Health Care, the availability of data and research has meant that we have been able to examine the role of women in medical practice and industrial issues for nurses. Of course these are just two of many issues that could have been examined to bring to light some of the issues surrounding women and health.

This book reflects many 'aortas' which have plagued most providers/educators trying to describe the area of women and health: it ought to be more brief, more detailed, more comparative, more women-centred, have more issues, have fewer issues. In short, more like mothers — everything to all people.

There are several chapters which serve as a starting point to a more general discussion but which really deserve a book on their own. An Historical Perspective — Women as Healers (chapter one) barely looks at the historical writings of some of the early women's health feminists, and An International Perspective — Women in Developing Countries (chapter two) is a summary of World Health Organization collated data. Chapters four (Women and Health Promotion) and 13 (Women and Ageing) are also only brushstrokes.

There are 'aortas' of exclusion too: it ought to be less American, less dated, less practical, less theoretical, less psychological, less medical and so on.

No single issue receives comprehensive coverage, for the book is meant as an introduction, not a definitive text.

The chapters in this book have been arranged around issues that are current for many women consumers and providers in Australia. However, most of those who seek professional help for health or social problems do not present as an 'issue'. They present as people with familes and jobs and hopes and fears. The case studies at the end of each chapter illustrate the ways in which clients may present to professionals, and the ways in which workers may respond to those they help. They do not describe a right or wrong way for providers or consumers to behave, react or respond. They are included to trigger thoughts and discussion about the complex issues that make up any one woman's life.

To reflect the real advances that can be achieved when women work together for change, this book is written from a woman-identified perspective. In an attempt to reverse the standard sexist language of our time we have followed Judith Lorber's example and used the pronoun 'she' in place of 'he'. Most researchers are deemed female. And this book is an example of women working together because it is not just the work of one author, but of several, some of whom contributed whole chapters, and all of whom contributed their knowledge, research, experiences, expertise and time.

Women consumers have become more vocal in expressing their health needs. Through a succession of institutional reviews of women's health, women consumers have made their needs be known loud and clear. In an effort to establish continuing validity for women's voices about health, the topic has had to be periodically redefined. The World Health Organization at its Decade of Women Conference in Nairobi gave it an international flavour and identified a set of strategies. The Women's Health Policy Review Committee Report (New South Wales) gave it 249 local flavours in the form of recommendations. Both reports identified the gross inequities in health as it relates to women as providers and consumers of health care. In 1989 *The National women's health policy: advancing women's health in Australia* was launched in response to mounting criticism that despite numerous reviews little action had taken place in this area.

However the best news is that women's health is no longer defined anatomically and enumerated in a series of impossible to achieve recommendations.

The policy promises to address the broadest context of women and health. Issues such as poverty, employment, access to educational opportunities, transport, housing, child care and sexist stereotyping in the media are mentioned in the last paragraph of the foreword. Unhappily however, as a framework for change, it falls far short of its espoused social model of health.

Australian based programs, designed for both providers and consumers, are needed. Initially these programs may have to deal with specific problems which are currently increasing women's morbidity: drug and alcohol addiction; body image and nutrition; occupational health of women workers; violence; and women with special needs. Focusing on these practical problems forces the closer examination of the role of women in society.

This shopping list of needs and demands is not unexpected. If you allow any oppressed group freedom of expression you can expect a morass of misery to be vocalised. Unfortunately, women are still dying from preventable causes, for example cervical cancer, before their needs are even recognised.

Unfortunately, too, Australian women have been educated into complicity. It is ironic that, despite numerous reviews of women's health, women consumers still have problems in ensuring that their needs are at least heard, let alone prioritised. Maybe, it's because the language is difficult to understand. All of these ideas require fundamental alterations in the nature of service provision in health care.

As providers, women have also been part of the double bind that affects all women who work in both paid and unpaid work. How can they be good health care providers if they don't work, or think work, 24 hours a day, seven days a week? How can they be good mothers if they do? Job-sharing, user-friendly part time rosters, wages and status-parity with full time health providers, and realistic retraining programs may be the answers to a broader medical malaise than just women's problems.

Injecting more women into the system is not the answer. In health care women already form the majority of providers. The real problem is that in terms of power and control they are still a minority. The short term result will be, as always, some of the more vocal complaints of women may be addressed through the writing of a report.

The structural issues raised by women consumers need more than passing attention. The range of health needs and problems of women, how we manage them, and the education of practitioners in these areas are important issues for our society.

Acknowledgments

This book developed out of two courses on Women and Health run as part of Masters programs at the University of New South Wales. Without the support of Professor Ian Webster and Frances Lovejoy these courses would never have surfaced. However, it is the postgraduate students, and their enthusiasm through the years, who have crystallised the ideas for this book. I would like to thank those students for their contribution. Thoughts alone do not make a book. Without the support and unending patience of my dear friend and publisher Jeremy Fisher this book would never have eventuated.

Many strong and beautiful women have supported me in my endeavours. Two are: Suzanne Donnolley, whose keyboard and editorial skills in the early phases were invaluable and overcame my professional illegibility; Gallia Therin, my memory, mentor and support person — we have been on many journeys together.

At a stage at which the completion of this book seemed impossible, along came Fiona Crawford, a highly intelligent foil to my flounderings. Her official title is editor but in this book she did much, much more than that title suggests. To her, great thanks. Thanks are also due to Rebecca Sheahan at Harcourt Brace Jovanovich who did a fine job with picture research.

Several chapters in this book would not have been possible without the generous efforts of my colleagues who have worked for many years in the area of women and health, often without recognition. In relation to specific chapters they are:

Dr Sally Redman, Senior Lecturer, School of Behavioural Sciences in Medicine, University of Newcastle, who wrote Chapter Three, Women's Major Health Needs and Chapter Seven, Women and Reproduction, and co-authored Chapter Eight, Women and Body Image;

Dr Jenny Barry, Sexual Assault Co-ordinator, South-Western Area of Sydney Health Service, who contributed to Chapter One, An Historical Perspective — Women as Healers, Chapter Nine, Women and Mental Health, and Chapter 11, Women and Violence;

Dr Andrea Mant, Senior Lecturer, School of Community Medicine, University of New South Wales, who contributed to Chapter Ten, Women and Substance Abuse;

Dr Carolyn Quadrio, Senior Lecturer, School of Psychiatry, University of New South Wales, who contributed to Chapter Six, Women and Sexuality;

Elizabeth Eglington, Senior Nurse Educator, Repatriation General Hospital, Concord, who contributed to Chapter Five, Women as Providers and Consumers of Health Care;

Peggy Trompf, Lecturer in Cross-cultural studies, School of Public Health, University of Sydney, who contributed to Chapter One, An Historical Perspective — Women as Healers and Chapter 13, Women with Special Needs;

Dr Susan Irvine, who wrote the case studies; and

Christine Paul, who researched Chapter Three, Women's Major Health Needs, Chapter Seven, Women and Reproduction, and Chapter Eight, Women and Body Image.

For the content and process of my life I would like to thank Lizzie and Marj.

Lastly, the Publisher and I wish to thank Professor Margaret Dunlop, Head, School of Nursing, Griffith University, who gave invaluable advice on the manuscript and proved to be a most astute reviewer.

Acknowledgments for Illustrations

p. 9, Sydney Hospital Library; p. 13, Mountford Oxford University Expedition, National Library of Australia; p. 19, Australian Associated Press; p. 26, United Nations High Commission for Refugees; p. 58, Cheryl McDonald, *A decade of change*, NSW Women's Advisory Council; p. 62, John Fairfax Group; p. 67, Royal Adelaide Hospital; p. 68, Maria Katrivesis, *A decade of change*, NSW Women's Advisory Council; p. 80, Carolyn Johns; p. 91, *The National Times*; p. 95, Abbott Diagnostics: a division of Abbott Australasia Pty Ltd; p. 98, Cheryl McDonald, *A decade of change*, NSW Women's Advisory Council; p. 106 (a), Wyeth Pharmaceuticals Pty Ltd; p. 106 (b), Abbott Australasia Pty Ltd; p. 114 (a) (b) (c), Berlei, a division of Pacific Dunlop Ltd; p. 122, Kerry Millard; p. 135, Margaret Olah; p. 151, Australian Dr Weekly; p. 158, Pamela Clements, *A decade of change*, NSW Women's Advisory Council; p. 167, Human Rights and Equal Opportunity Commission; p. 174, Margaret Olah; p. 178, Margaret Olah; p. 188, Margaret Olah; p. 191, Margaret Olah; p. 203, John Fairfax Group.

The author and publishers have made every effort to contact the owners of copyright work used in this volume. However, should such work have been reproduced without permission, correction will be made in future printings.

1 An Historical Perspective
— Women As Healers

This chapter explores the role of women in health care in European and Australian history. Historically, women's role as providers of health care has been ignored, devalued or radically suppressed. Definitive writings date from the beginning of the twentieth century. In Australia the written history of women in health care is limited to a European focus and the history of Aboriginal women as health providers has largely been ignored. It is vital to examine and explore the past in order to understand the current status quo.

Throughout history women have played a basic and essential role in the provision of health care. There have been concerted attempts by individuals and groups of women to question the status quo as prescribed by the Church and/or State. These movements have ranged from arguing for a better deal at the hands of a male-dominated medical world to demanding and taking full responsibility for their own and other women's health.

ANCIENT HISTORY

Women have been involved in health care since ancient times. In many primitive societies men hunted for food while women were responsible, as a natural addition to their gathering of plants, seeds and roots, for the health care needs of their communities, learning to use plant and other substances in a variety of remedies.

Mary Chamberlain (1981) asserts that up to 3000 BC, in ancient Egypt, Greece and Assyria, healing was almost exclusively the domain of priestesses. The separate occupation of midwifery was also an exclusively female concern. Concepts of illness were linked inextricably to prevailing cultural and religious beliefs and as these values changed, the power of the priestesses was eroded and male healing deities began to emerge. Around 3000 BC the first male physician was appointed to the Egyptian court. Chamberlain suggests that the ascent of male physicians saw increased use of surgery and a reduction in the less invasive healing practices favoured by the priestess physicians.

Although women continued to play a role in health care at the family level, Lyons and Petrucelli (1979) imply that history only records as important in health care provision such eminent names as Hippocrates, credited with the earliest recorded attempt to scientifically separate medicine from superstition.

JUDEO-CHRISTIAN ERA

The rise of Christianity crystallised social attitudes to women and women healers. Women were likened to Eve, the original sinner and essentially evil. Morally and intellectually they were excluded from religious practice. Divinity and disease became inter-related. St. Mark refers to Jesus Christ's first healing act as the 'tearing out of an unclean spirit' (1: 23-27), equating sickness with sin. Spiritually inferior to men, women were thus considered unfit to attend the sick. In some areas, however, women were permitted to practise midwifery, provided they recognised that they were ultimately answerable to God and to his earthly representatives, priests. The attitude of the early Christians towards women, combined with their ignorance of the causation of disease and illness, made women perfect scapegoats. They were seen as 'witches', capable of casting spells and causing disease. Medical care, as practised by the male physicians, was really only available to the higher classes, leaving the majority of people to fend for themselves and to rely upon folk remedies and similar practices. Chamberlain's findings (1981) agree with those of Lyons and Petrucelli (1979). She points out that:

> The poor had little choice but to continue with home remedies and unorthodox practitioners. This duality of medical practice remained a feature of European medicine until the twentieth century.

The practice of medicine remained strongly linked to religion, with Claudius Galen (c129-c200) systemising medical knowledge according to his ideas of creation by the will of God. He believed in the existence of teleological explanations for everything. Lyons and Petrucelli (1979) believe that Galen's view that nature (God) must have given a clear purpose to all functions and organs deluded him into distorting what he saw. Galen's influence was to last more than 1000 years.

JEWISH WOMEN IN HEALTH CARE

The visible removal of women from the conduct of Jewish religious life has led to erroneous assumptions about the role of women within the context of their Jewish societies. Goitein (1973) in her discussion of Jewish women in the middle ages suggests that whilst Talmudic law placed restrictions on women within the Jewish religious culture, the role of women within their societies was not always limited or hidden. Henry and Taitz (1983) discovered that Jewish women led full lives in the middle ages in places like Egypt and in the Mediterranean communities. Documents of the Cairo Geniza reveal that Jewish women worked as midwives, doctors, teachers in girls' schools, undertakers or textile merchants.

Amongst the Jews who fled from the Spanish Inquisition to find refuge in Italian cities during the 15th and 16th centuries were many women committed to health care studies. Roth (1959) records the work of a woman physician named Perna who was licensed in 1460 in Fano, Italy. Her role was limited. Roth suggests that women physicians in Italy most likely attended only women, despite the freer access of all Jewish physicians to Arabic medicine which made the Jewish male physicians increasingly popular amongst heads of state and even Popes.

From the ghettos of Europe in the 17th and 18th centuries came a new movement in Judaism called Hasidism which changed the religious self image of the average Jew by introducing the idea that one's emotional response to God is equally, if not more important, than religious study. Within this context Jewish women thrived both in religious and secular life.

Ghettos in some ways shielded Jewish communities from developments in the countries in which they lived. However, the developments in professionalisation of medical practice and the marginalisation of women into reproductive work, determined the course of all women healers in Europe.

MIDDLE AGES — RENAISSANCE

Ehrenreich and English (1973a) describe the conflict between the traditional healing wisdom of women and male expertise centered on the right to heal. Across all classes the art of healing was linked to the tasks of motherhood. All women were expected to understand herbs and healing techniques. The systematic examination of healing which became the profession of medicine excluded all but the most privileged of women.

The establishment of medical schools began in Europe in the 11th century, with the first of these at Salerno in Italy. However, with the exception of the Italian schools, women were not admitted. Women graduates are recorded from Salerno, including Trotula, a woman physician reputed to be the author of the first obstetrics and gynaecology textbook. A few other women, mostly from the upper classes, were able to achieve fame as healers and to leave some record of their work and beliefs.

As medicine professionalised and became male and expensive, the bulk of health care for the poor was delivered by women healers. Women made up virtually all of the midwives and formed a large percentage of the 'unorthodox practitioners' or empirical healers. Ironically, the empirical healers' practices were often more successful than those of the educated, mostly male physicians. Blum (1974) rediscovers *Liber Simplicis Medicinae,* St Hildegarde of Bingen's book in which she describes the properties of 213 varieties of plants and trees, which were known to have healing properties. Jewett (1972) outlines how testimonials as to the power of women's healing practices extended across continents and centuries. The other major group of women to work with the sick poor were nuns, who provided refuge, nourishment and sometimes, specific cures, to those in their care.

Women healers, or 'wise women' and 'old wives', as they were known, handed on their knowledge from mother to daughter over many generations. Unlike their socially acceptable brothers, the women did not have access to books and derived little monetary benefit from their skills. However, much of their expertise was the empiric research on which medical theories were based. Many of the herbs used by women, e.g. Foxglove or digitalis as it is now called, were incorporated into the repertoire of current medical knowledge by observant academics, who now claim the tablet as their own.

The attitudes towards and styles of health care practised by the women healers differed markedly from those of the academic physicians. These differences are illustrated in the case of Jacoba Felicie, reported by Ehrenreich and English (1973*b*). In around 1322 Felicie, a skilled Parisian healer, was charged with illegal practice on the following counts:

- visiting the sick at home
- feeling the pulse, checking the urine and touching the limbs of the sick
- making up cures
- regularly visiting to check on the progress of the sick
- accepting a fee

Called as witnesses at her trial, her patients applauded her skills, comparing her expertise very favourably with that of the physicians, with whom they had had less beneficial encounters. In her defence, Felicie pleaded the need for women to be visited by women doctors on the grounds of modesty, but to no avail. She was found guilty of the charges and forbidden to practise medicine in or near Paris. Her crime, it would seem, was to encroach on the territory of the 'trained' physicians and to beat them at their own game. Had she remained working among the poor, then her work would have remained largely ignored, like that of thousands of other practising women healers.

The male physicians' reaction to the threat of the women healers did not limit itself to trials such as Felicie's. Supported by Church and State, these early 'professionals' colluded in a strategic campaign of terror which was to span almost four centuries — the notorious witch hunts which spread throughout Europe from the 14th to the 17th centuries.

The German monks Kramer and Sprenger (1484), according to Chamberlain (1981), established the witch hunt in their infamous *Malleus Maleficarium* (Hammer of Witches). ('Malleus' is a hammer, firebrand or axe used to fell an animal about to be sacrificed and 'maleficarium' means 'power to work harm'.) Witches were accused of working harm through such means as: having magical powers affecting health for better or for worse; being organised; and committing every conceivable crime against men.

Ehrenreich and English (1973b) suggest that the inquisitors reserved their greatest wrath for the midwives, who, they claimed, committed the greatest injuries to the Faith. This assertion was based on confessions obtained from some of the women, before they were burned at the stake.

If women had the power to cure illness, then, it was argued, they also had the power to cause it. According to the Church, the poor became sick because sickness was clearly the result of sinning. Salvation was obtainable only through suffering and prayer. Certainly, they should not seek help at the hands of the wise women and midwives, who were now reclassified as heretics and 'witches'.

But how could anyone tell if an illness was caused by witchcraft? Kramer and Sprenger came up with an ingenious solution:

If it is asked how it is possible to distinguish whether an illness is caused by witchcraft or by some other natural defect, we answer that the first (way) is by means of the judgement of doctors.

Thus, the final arbiter became the male physicians, the group whose power had been most threatened by the skills of the women midwives and healers.

Michelet (1939), Murray (1921), Hole (1957), Kors and Peters (1972), and Hughes (1952) all give graphic accounts of the magnitude and implications of the witch hunts. During the course of the witch hunts, thousands and possibly millions of women were burned at the stake or otherwise killed. Ehrenreich and English (1973b) conclude that more than 85 per cent of the victims were women and in some communities almost no adult women were left alive. Although the reasons for the witch hunts have been linked to other broad social developments, such as the Reformation, the rise of commerce, increasingly frequent uprisings against the aristocracy etc, it cannot be ignored that the targets were mostly peasant women, who were predominantly midwives and lay healers Although not totally eliminated as a result of the witch hunts, women healers and midwives became discredited and treated with suspicion.

With the decline of witches as legitimate health providers came the abandonment of the notion of supernatural causes for mental and physical ill health. In the seventeenth century the death penalty for witchcraft was abolished in France.

Throughout this time the medical schools flourished in Europe, turning out male physicians who were becoming increasingly accepted as the only legitimate practitioners of healing as 'scientific medicine'. Lyons and Petrucelli suggest that as teaching in medical schools was controlled by the Church, the study of medicine was concerned largely with the explanation of medicine and nature through theology as Galen had predestined. However, most of the practical knowledge was derived from 'wise women'. In fact, Theophrastus Bombastus von Hohenheim, or Paracelsus (1565), admitted that he had gained all his medical knowledge from the 'sorceress'.

SIXTEENTH TO EIGHTEENTH CENTURY

During the 17th century, formal health provider structures and professional organisations for male surgeons, physicians, dentists and apothecaries were developed. These were the basis for the modern Royal Colleges. It was impossible, however, for women to be accepted for training and practice as doctors. Italy continued to be the only exception. In that country, women occupied prestigious university chairs.

Although the male art of surgery was flourishing, male attendants were rarely present at the birth of children. Rowbotham (1973) asserts that conception and childbirth in the early 19th century were 'seditious and blasphemous' topics for working class women. However, by the early 18th century it became fashionable, in certain parts of Europe, for middle and upper class women to have a male attendant during childbirth. This period saw the introduction of obstetric forceps. Women were further marginalised in perinatal care, when increasing concern was voiced by male doctors about wetnurses supposedly transmitting infectious diseases between babies. In England, Elizabeth Cellier was instrumental in the establishment of a special hospital for women. She was later pilloried for her criticisms of obstetric practices.

NINETEENTH TO EARLY TWENTIETH CENTURY

With increasing industrialisation and urbanisation, the role of the midwife and wise woman underwent further change. She became less integral to the small communities which had once sustained her.

By the early 1800s there were many male 'regular' doctors who had undergone formal training in medical schools. They went to great lengths to distinguish themselves from the lay practitioners. As a result of these social changes, they had become increasingly involved in treating the ordinary classes. Thus, increasing numbers of people were experiencing the remedies which relied on both scientific advances in the areas of infection control and empiric and often 'heroic' measures such as bloodletting, purging (including vomiting, using laxatives and enemas) and the production of blisters using, for example, mustard plaster. Ehrenreich and English (1979) assert that, although these remedies were labelled as scientific (and therefore should have been based on sound principles of inquiry and evaluation), they were used quite indiscriminately and arbitrarily.

In the United States of America, in particular, outrage against the seemingly indiscriminate use of medical practices and regular medicines led to a mass movement against medical professionalism. Hurd-Mead, in 1938, formalised the so-called Popular Health Movement which arose out of feminist and working class movements of the late nineteenth and early twentieth centuries. The emphasis of this movement was on preventive health care, education and sharing of information, dietary changes and the judicious use of herbs. The women's groups, including such notable women as Fanny Wright in the US, organised benevolent associations, charitable institutions, courses in health care for women and mutual support groups.

These groups flourished for half a century but gradually began to demand recognition and status akin to that demanded by the regular doctors they had criticised. Meanwhile, as with the knowledge of the wise women before, the regular doctors had begun to incorporate into their own practices some of the principles of the Popular Health Movement.

Women, however, continued to speak out against the excesses of the heroic measures used by the 'regular' doctors. They also revived a much earlier concern, the specific nature of the male doctor-female patient relationship. Many felt that their energies ought to be directed at supporting women who wanted to enter medical school and become doctors. The provision of more women doctors was seen as the solution to the problems women were suffering at the hands of male doctors. In 1849 Elizabeth Blackwell graduated as the first woman regular doctor in the US. It would be nearly thirty-five years before Australia would accept its first female medical student. Blackwell quickly discovered how difficult her task was. Throughout her career she continued to struggle against various forms of discrimination. For example, Leeson and Grey (1978) maintain that the Professor of Gynaecology at St Bartholomew's in London would not allow her to study 'his subject' . This particular situation pertains today in regard to women who wish to pursue this speciality (see chapter five).

NURSING

Florence Nightingale, a member of the British upper classes, organised a band of 38 'gentlewomen volunteers' to act as nurses during the Crimean War (1850s). Using commonsense and discipline, as well as an understanding of the importance of cleanliness she was able to dramatically reduce the death rate on the front from 50 per cent to a mere 2 per cent. Nightingale summed up women's longstanding role in health care as follows:

> every woman, or at least almost every woman ... has, at one time or another of her life, charge of the health of somebody, whether child or invalid — in other words, every woman is a nurse (Nightingale 1969).

She also pointed out that the work of the nurse differed from that of the housemaid only in so far as it included attending to the sick. The art of nursing was based on two principles. The first of these was hygiene. Nightingale strongly believed that lack of sanitation was the major cause of ill health. This was more than just a connection between dirt and disease, but the belief that 'filth was the nexus of moral failing and sickness. Cleanliness was simultaneously a moral and hygienic imperative' (Holton 1984). Disease represented moral failure, with hygiene becoming an almost religious observance. Nursing constituted a 'calling' — a worldly vocation, but one which required the same degree of self sacrifice as did the religious orders. In addition to strict hygiene, Nightingale (1969) insisted that nursing required 'the proper use of fresh air, light, warmth, cleanliness, quiet, selection and administration of diet — all at the least expense to the patient'.

The second function of nursing was that of maidservant to the doctor. Here, obedience was the primary virtue of the nurse. Nurses should not see themselves as colleagues or advisors to doctors, but rather as handmaidens. The doctor could thus be freed the tedium of bedside care and maximise all his academic training in diagnosis and treatment planning. Nursing was seen as a feminine role, based on service and sacrifice, and, as described by Leeson and Grey (1978), 'an extension of the "natural function" of women as help-mate to the men doctors' .

The probationer nurse in the 1850s signed an agreement that placed her under the regulation and direction of the hospital and training school for five years. Surveillance and regimentation even extended to what she wore outside work and where she lived.

Nightingale argued for nurses to be adequately trained, but once training was accepted as a method of getting good nursing staff, the qualities looked for and concentrated upon were caring rather than curative. The former were the feminine domain of nurses, the latter consigned to the higher realm of male doctors. This only served to reinforce the patriarchal relationship between men and women in accepting a division of labour which supported ideas of men's work and women's work on traditional grounds. Many aspects of nurses' work became identified with domestic labour and many analogies developed between nursing and motherhood. The following statement was made in 1897.

The best nurse is that woman whose maternal instincts are well developed ... the connection between mothering and nursing is very close (Gamarnikow 1978).

Compare those sentiments with these, expressed in 1976 by John Harrington, Barrister for the Australian Health Commission '...Your honour, to be against nurses is to be against motherhood and the flag ...'

NURSING IN AUSTRALIA

Best (1988), in his book, *Portraits in Australian Health*, documents Australian nursing history.

Nursing in Australia formally commenced with the construction of the first hospital in February 1788. A small hut located on the west side of Sydney Cove was surrounded by tents each holding four patients. Initially accommodating sixty, then over eighty patients, it was moved to Dawes Point in 1796. By 1806 there were some 5000 sick in the colony.

The hospital was staffed by five female nurses paid 40 pounds a year. They were mostly elderly women recruited from amongst the colony's domestic servants and from the general population. They had no training and were uneducated and illiterate. Their experience was acquired in the wards. Male patients were nursed entirely by male nurses who were recruited from discharged patients.

The first trained nurses in Australia were a group of five Sisters of Charity nuns who arrived from Ireland in 1838. They began their work at the women's penitentiary at Parramatta. In 1840, the Sisters of Charity opened a hospital at Potts Point which introduced new nursing methods. Later, in 1858, the Sisters opened St Vincent's Hospital with Mother Baptist de Lacy in charge.

Professional training for nurses began in Australia in the early 1860s at the Lying-in Hospital at Carlton in Victoria, which subsequently became the Royal Women's Hospital, Melbourne. Although some instruction in nursing was available at the hospital from the time it was opened in 1856, the first formal training of nurses began in 1861/62.

The first school for training nurses opened in Sydney in 1868, following a written request in 1866 by Prime Minister, Sir Henry Parkes to Florence Nightingale. His aim was to enlist her assistance in a scheme to introduce trained nurses to the colony. The Nightingale Training School for nurses at St Thomas' Hospital in London had opened six years earlier. Her plan was to 'train nurses to train' and then send them abroad. Miss Nightingale responded and after negotiations approved the Parkes scheme.

Miss Lucy Osburn, in the position of Lady Superintendent, accompanied by five English nursing sisters, sailed to Australia, arriving in Sydney in March 1868. They immediately took up duties at Sydney Hospital, enacting regulations and affecting reforms. Miss Osburn had full responsibility for the nursing and the internal management of the wards at Sydney Hospital. Male nursing positions were abolished.

By 1873 the nursing staff of Sydney Hospital comprised four head-nurses and seventeen nurses and probationers. All of the nurses, except for one from the original group of five, had been trained at the hospital. In 1884, Miss Osburn retired and her successor, Miss McKay, became the first Australian-trained nurse to hold the position of matron. The earliest appointment of a certified matron was a Miss Turiff at the newly-erected Alfred Hospital in Melbourne.

In Tasmania, Hobart Hospital set up a school in 1875. The Children's Hospital in Melbourne began a training course for pupil nurses in 1878 and professional training of nurses began at the Homeopathic Hospital (later renamed Prince Henry Hospital) and the Ballarat and District Base Hospital in 1885. In New South Wales, training schools for nurses at the Royal Prince Alfred and St Vincent's hospitals date from 1882.

Training schools flourished, each with different training programs and length of service requirements. In 1887 regulations were introduced which required all trainees to undergo a regular course of instruction which extended over two years. A certificate was granted on completion of the course and after passing the necessary examinations.

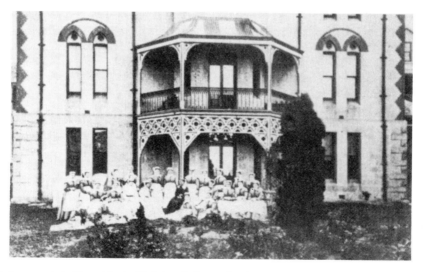

Lucy Osburn and staff outside the Nightingale Wing of Sydney Hospital

Further to this initial regulation, a group of Nurse Administrators established the Australian Trained Nurses Association (ATNA) in Sydney in 1899. The ATNA took over the registration of training schools, the examination of trainees and the registration of nurses. The first examination under the ATNA was held in 1906.

Nurses were performing a general bedside role in patients' homes, in the small district hospitals and the larger city hospitals. This role was extended to the scattered inland population by the foundation of the Bush Nursing Society in 1911.

From this time on, women's 'legitimate' role in health care developed along a variety of paths. With increasing government regulations, licensing laws and Acts of Parliament determining who can do what, women have ended up working in a number of differing health care 'occupations', each jealously guarding its own 'territory'. Others have chosen to work outside these 'occupations'.

TWENTIETH CENTURY

By the early part of this century, increasing numbers of women were accepted into the medical profession. Unfortunately, this has had little impact on the training experienced by doctors. Many women doctors are as elitist and exploitative as the men their forebears criticised, while others continue to suffer discrimination similar to that experienced by Elizabeth Blackwell.

In 1902 in the UK, the profession of midwifery was regulated by an Act of Parliament. Concerted campaigns resulted in the virtual demise of this group in the US and Australia. Even in the UK, the number of midwives is now declining with increasing numbers of births in hospitals. By 1919 nursing had also become a regulated profession in the UK. Feminists such as Margaret Sanger, Emma Goldman (both nurses) and Marie Stopes began to speak out in relation to women controlling their bodies. Each of these women suffered persecution and discrimination because of her outspokenness and commitment.

Since the Second World War, the number of women in the health professions has escalated, mostly in the so called 'ancillary' roles (from the Latin 'ancilla', meaning handmaid) of nurse, social worker, physiotherapist, occupational therapist, dietitian, speech therapist etc.

The Coffs Harbour Women's Health Centre

In 1973, 17 women met to found the Coffs Harbour branch of Cowper Women's Electoral Lobby. When the Decade for Women began two years later, WEL was already lobbying on a number of issues with considerable vigour. During that decade, enormous growth took place among local women, both at personal and community level. Changes in attitudes were profound and there is no doubt that the impetus for change was initiated by WEL.

In 1975, WEL brought to Coffs Harbour the YWCA photographic exhibition *Woman in celebration of International Women's Year*. In 150 pictures were captured the joys, grief, dignity and humiliation of women and their struggle for affirmation and the maintenance of their identity.

It was WEL that researched the need and was basically responsible for the establishment of a women's refuge and a family planning unit. In some sections of the community, there were cries of rage and disbelief that such places were considered necessary in their town, but in 1978 Warrina Women's Refuge opened its door and has operated at full capacity ever since. By the end of the Decade for Women, it had long had community respect and acceptance.

By 1982, WEL had encouraged a small group of feminists to open a women's resource centre. At first unfunded, it later received a Wage Pause grant and a CEP grant, enabling employment of salaried co-ordinators and project officers.

Through the resource centre, women were introduced to the concepts of self-help and networking. Of vital importance in the educative process were regular weekend workshops, centred around guest speakers drawn from feminists prominent in a number of spheres. Women's dinners were a feature of these occasions and rapidly increased in popularity, providing a relaxed atmosphere in which women could meet, talk and listen. During 1983 WEL was absorbed into the resource centre.

Despite a quite aggressive smear campaign against its formation, the family planning unit was achieved in the middle of 1984. It was based at the Community Health Centre. By then, planning for a women's Health Centre was under way.

Early in 1985, the now internationally known Women for Health came into being, to intensify the urgent investigation into the spraying of agricultural chemicals in the area. It was co-ordinated by two members of the Women's Resource Centre. Later in that year, women in the community were invited to contribute to the planning of the health centre. Their enthusiasm, energy, ideas and support were given abundantly at unforgettable meetings of enormous vitality. The dream that had started within a small group of women was soon to become a reality for many.

Early in 1986, Coffs Harbour Women's Health Centre was opened and just as WEL had allowed itself to be absorbed by the resource centre, so the resource centre was absorbed into the health centre. A quiet beginning had been expected, perhaps a period when the community might need encouragement to overcome some diffidence about using the new resource. That didn't happen. Within hours of opening, the service was booked out for three months ahead. It had not been realised how ready women were, how the decade had prepared them for the concept of women caring for themselves.

The health centre offers a gynaecological unit of two medical practitioners, a nurse practitioner conducting a Well Women's Health Clinic, counselling, natural therapies, such as acupuncture, herbalism and massage, along with home birth support. As well, the family planning clinic is now operating within the Health Centre.

Educative programs explore issues of empowerment and physical and psychological well being. Child care is provided and there is an ever expanding library from which clients may borrow books. The centre is funded at State level by the Department of Health.

Three women have commented on the centre:

'I felt I should have a smear test, but hated the thought of going to a male doctor. The idea of a women's health centre just seemed so good to me. I went there with hormonal problems and the threat of a hysterectomy looming, an operation I didn't want, but was being pushed towards. The women's centre was my last hope and they were wonderful. They keep trying. They never give up on you. They keep listening until they discover what's causing your problem.

'To be quite honest, all that other doctors had offered as a solution to my problems was valium and I didn't want it. If the women's health centre hadn't been there, I'm sure I'd have gone under. I go there knowing I'll be helped, not treated as though I'm stupid.'

'I thought possibly I'd experience more empathy about women's complaints from a woman doctor. I felt perhaps there'd be a more intuitive approach by a woman. I was absolutely right about that: empathy, the intuitive approach and the feeling that they cared, they were concerned.'

In Coffs Harbour and district, women achieved much during the Decade for Women. From the initial experience of WEL, they moved out into other organisations, spread their growing skills, learnt to use the media, talked, listened, changed, grew, encouraged other women to do the same.

From *A decade of change, women in New South Wales 1976–86*, NSW Women's Advisory Council to the Premier.

WOMEN AS HEALERS IN TRADITIONAL ABORIGINAL SOCIETY

Health for Aborigines is according to the National Aboriginal Health Strategy 1989 a:

> matter of determining all aspects of their life, including control over their physical environment, of dignity, of community self esteem and of justice. It is not merely a matter of the provision of doctors, hospitals, medicines or the absence of disease and incapacity.

There is no expression or word, as westerners understand, for 'health' in Aboriginal culture, which would not make sense of 'health' as just one aspect of life. Rather, as in other ideas of holistic medicine (Chinese systems for example), the term might best be translated into something which means, as suggested by the National Aboriginal Health Strategy, 'life is health in life'.

The integrality of health to life is explained by the

> traditional Aboriginal social systems (which) include a 3 dimensional model that provides a blue print for living (and) is based on interrelationships between people and land, people and creator beings, and between people, which ideally stipulates inter-dependence within and between each set of relationships (National Aboriginal Health Strategy).

Gordon Briscoe (1978) notes the traditional social structure was 'probably the most important factor which enabled Aboriginal groups to effectively control the level of their own health...'. This social structure incorporates a 'health consciousness' which traditionally functions through an authority structure comprised of clever men or women. Briscoe writes 'in rural communities of the eastern seaboard it functions similarly through the dominant women figures ...'

Earlier anthropologists and other commentators on Aboriginal society presented a male-centred view of the society. Thus scholars such as Elkin (1945, 1954) wrote in the masculine when discussing traditional Aboriginal healers. We know now that women also were and are capable of being 'clever'. Describing the functions of medicine men, Elkin discusses their life giving properties:

> he restores life by getting rid of sickness, or by recapturing the straying soul: he is the link with the unseen spirit world and the sky from which life is obtained, and he can ascertain the causes of illness and death (1954).

The Aboriginal doctor is part of a system of social control in that he or she influences behaviour, and is committed to producing a desirable behavioural change in the patient. Thus medicine and the law are synthesised to the extent that there are some common procedures for healing and for the maintenance of social order (Soong 1983).

Traditionally, it appears that women took a more dominant role in the performance of healing rituals. Dianne Bell (1983) notes that women's ceremonies were concentrated on major life events — birth, menarche and death. The rituals were concerned in one way or another with the health of the community. Bell writes

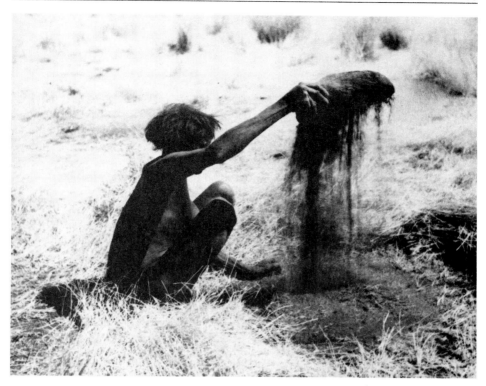

Aboriginal woman winnowing seeds

'women as the ritual nurturers of relationships seek to maintain and to restore harmony, happiness and thus health.'

Bell (1983), in her study of the Walbiri people of Central Australia discusses the way in which a woman becomes a Ngangkayi or healer. Women in this role perform health maintenance activities, through ritual performance, and also in the application of healing substances. However, this is essentially 'an individual activity concerned more with the removal of foreign objects and alien forces from a person'.

Women in general are widely involved in health maintenance which extends beyond the use of herbal remedies and the care of children. Women stage ceremonies

> which focus on health at the right cosmic level of restoration of harmony and happiness. This is because women have rights in the country from which they derive power and for which they hold a sacred trust ... All women's groups ritual curing activities have to do with giving — with the infusing of the body with strength ... In giving, women ... once again are acting out their nurturance role where love, care and power are freely given.

This theme is reiterated by other observers (Munn 1973; Hamilton 1981). For the Walbiri, there is a difference between ways men and women contribute to the maintenance of the Dreaming, and hence the maintenance of a whole or healthy society. The feminine role

is focussed in the personal, biological and family plane of life maintenance. The part women play in ritual (including their role in men's initiation rites) and the major functions of their own ancestral designs tend to be confined to such matters as female sexuality, personal health, and the growth of children (Munn 1973).

Women's business

There were and are still areas of health that are known only to mature women. The secrecy surrounding this knowledge is quite profound and even as late as 1975 it was seen as being 'difficult to obtain accurate information about what is regarded as women's business, although menstruation, miscarriage and pregnancy fall into

Aboriginal birth in the bush

This is the story ...

When a mother is pregnant, she is not allowed to eat big things like emu, barramundi, cod, big crabs, kangaroo, big goanna, stingray, barla, crocodile, brown water snake or big sugar boy (that's wild honey). When mother is seven months she is not allowed to sleep with her husband because it will be very hard for her when she goes into labour. Well, in our society, for a traditional way of giving birth, the mother is taken to a deeper part of the bush, with the grandmother and the mother-in-law where there is no wind and ants and people cannot see. The ground is dug half deep: the mother sits with her bottom half way up and her knees firmly apart. The grandmother sits in front, to see the baby doesn't fall in the dirt. The mother-in-law, she sits at the back of her daughter-in-law to see she has a lot of balance: she is not to give a push until her mother-in-law tells her to do so. When baby arrives the mother-in-law sits in front to pull the cord. Then all tribal names are called and when the whole part comes out we have that name we call 'Thapich'. After mother is cleaned up and they put mother in a good comfortable humpy where she is well looked after and properly fed.

Baby is put in a Gan. It's a bark basket of teatree bark. Teatree was also our blankets as well as our clothes. If the mother has no milk in the breast, well the grandmother hunts for a young milkwood tree, pulls the young leaf and draws three lines on the breast, and suddenly the breast is full of milk. The mother's foods are still the same until the time when the baby is strong, turns on his or her tummy and the second skin is changed. Then preparations are made by the grandparents for the mother to be put in for strengthening. The mother and the baby are painted with paint. The mother is pressed against the Iron Wood Tree with her legs open over a fire that is made near the trunk of the tree. When we throw water on the fire we believe that smoke goes in to the womb and we press a stone tomahawk on the tummy. Then the mother and baby are taken by parents to meet the proud father and uncles. Baby is dressed with paint and feathers and father carries netbag, spears and warm mar. Father proudly puts smell from his underarm onto baby and bites the baby so he or she could be strong. But this doesn't mean Daddy can sleep with Mummy (no) until her womb is strong after the first period. Then he can sleep with Mummy.

We have medicines we can take to have baby or not to have baby, and to make mother have plenty of milk. When the baby has plenty of teeth, mother is allowed big meat or fish.

Joyce Hall (an Aboriginal woman from North Queensland), *New doctor* (1980), 15, 44.

this category' (Connor 1975). In fact much of women's business deals with female sexuality and reproduction.

Aboriginal women have traditionally given birth according to the Grandmother Alukura Law ('alukura' means a place to give birth). As an Aboriginal woman put it

> for us, pregnancy, childbirth and postnatal care have always been women's business, according to our Women's Law. We have our own Traditional Birth attendants and practices ... Our traditional beliefs and practices are anchored in the Dreamtime and the Law. They are radically different to western beliefs and practices. Birth is not just an act of labour but is used to refer to a much wider and more symbolic process. It begins at conception in a particular area of country and is inseparable from the Dreamtime, and the Law and the people, resulting in strong traditional affiliations, rights and responsibilities to that country. The labouring woman is attended by Traditional Birth attendants (women skilled and knowledgable in the Law who might be her Grandmother, Aunt, older sister) by a fire to make it warm for mother and baby according to our Grandmother Alukura Law. Afterwards special ceremonies are performed by those same women. The women also help her on a day to day basis in caring for herself and her baby (Abbott 1985).

CASE STUDY

It was in 1969 that a group of women in Boston calling themselves 'the doctors' group' met to discuss health issues and to share their feelings of frustration and disenfranchisement with the American medical system, which they felt was male dominated, insensitive and paternalistic, with regard to matters of women's reproductive health. These women were mostly middle class, well educated working mothers in their twenties and thirties. They used many methods to learn more about topics which interested them — childbirth, contraception, sexuality, anatomy — and then they shared their learning with one another. To have such knowledge to share and build on was exciting and exhilarating, and a more structured educational format developed. A year later after a second course a newsprint edition of their discussions was published and distributed in Boston for 75 cents. This included personal comments by women who had taken the courses, and was entitled *Women and Their Bodies*. Within two years 250,000 copies had been sold, and it was clear that there was a deeply felt need by American women to know and understand their own bodies. So the Boston Women's' Health Book Collective was formed, with a membership of twelve, and in 1972 *Our Bodies, Ourselves*, was published for the mass market. It achieved phenomenal success, became a best seller, has gone into many printings, and nearly twenty languages, and is now in its third edition.

All that from the efforts of a small group of women. Their dedication and commitment extended the impact of the book beyond its educational and informational impact. It began the process of recognising that nearly all women shared feelings of powerlessness and helplessness, about their reproductive function, and showed that change in health for women does not take place only in a doctor's surgery, but in publishing houses, in academic institutions, in political arenas, and above all when women tap their own abilities allowing themselves the freedom and the confidence to explore their own bodies, and their own feelings and fears and dreams.

REFERENCES

Abbott, L. (1985). The central Australian Aboriginal Congress birthright research and birthrights program, *Women's health in a changing society,* proceedings of the 2nd national conference on all aspects of women's health, Adelaide, September, vol. 2.

Bell, D. (1983). *Daughters of the dreaming,* McPhee Gribble, Sydney.

Best, J. (1988). *Portraits in Australian health,* MacLennan and Petty, Sydney.

Blum, S.B. (1974). Women witches and herbals, *The Morris Arboretum bulletin,* 25, 43.

Briscoe, G. (1978). Aboriginal health and land rights, *New doctor,* 8, 13–15.

Chamberlain, M. (1981). *Old wives tales: their history, remedies and spells,* Virago Press, London.

Connor, A. (1975). Family planning among Aborigines, *The medical journal of Australia,* special supplement, vol. 1, no. 3.

Ehrenreich, B. & English, D. (1973*a*). *Complaints and disorders: the sexual politics of sickness,* Writers and Readers Publishing Co-operative, London.

Ehrenreich B. & English D. (1973*b*). *Witches, midwives and nurses,* The Feminist Press, London.

Ehrenreich, B. & English, D. (1979). *For her own good,* Pluto Press, London.

Elkin, A.P. (1945). *Aboriginal men of high degree,* University of Queensland Press, St Lucia.

Elkin, A.P. (1954). *The Australian Aborigines: how to understand them,* 3rd ed., Angus & Robertson, Sydney.

Gamarnikow, E. (1978). *Sexual division of labour: the case of nursing,* WHO Nos, Sydney.

Goitein, S. D. (1973). New revelations from the Cairo Geniza: Jewish women in the middle ages, *Hadassah magazine,* October, 14–15.

Hamilton, A. (1981). *Nature and nurture: Aboriginal child rearing in North Central Arnhem,* Australian Institute of Aboriginal Studies, Canberra.

Harrington, J. (1976). *The Lamp,* May.

Henry, S. & Taitz, E. (1983). *Written out of history: our Jewish foremothers,* Biblio Press, Fresh Meadows NY.

Hole, C. (1957). *A mirror of witchcraft,* Chatto and Windus, London.

Holton, S. (1984). *Feminine authority and social order: Florence Nightingale's conception of nursing and health care,* Virago, London.

Hughes, P. (1952). *Witchcraft,* Penguin Books, London.

Hurd-Mead, K.C. (1938). *A history of women in medicine,* Haddam, Connecticut.

Jewett, S.O. (1972). The courting of Sister Wisby, in G. Parker (ed.) *The oven birds: American women on womanhood 1820–1920.* Doubleday/Achor, New York.

Kors, A.C. & Peters, E. (1972). *Witchcraft in Europe: 1100–1700,* University of Pennsylvania Press, Philadelphia.

Leeson, J. & Grey, J. (1978). *Women and medicine,* Tavistock Publications, London.

Lyons A.S. & Petrucelli R.J. (1979). *Medicine — an illustrated history,* Macmillan, South Melbourne.

Michelet, J. (1939). *Satanism and witchcraft,* Citadel Press, New Jersey.

Munn, N. (1973). *Walbiri iconography,* Cornell University Press, Ithaca.

Murray, M.A. (1921). *The witch cult in western Europe,* Oxford University Press, New York.

National Aboriginal health strategy working party (1989). National Aboriginal health strategy.

Nightingale, F. (1969). *Notes on nursing. What it is and what it is not,* Dover Publications, New York.

Roth C. (1959). *The Jews in the Renaissance,* Jewish Publication Society of America, Philadelphia.

Rowbotham, S. (1976). *Hidden from history: rediscovering women in history from 17th century to the present,* Pluto Press, London.

Soong, F.S. (1983). Role of the Margidjbu (traditional healer) in western Arnhem land, *The medical journal of Australia,* 1, 474–7.

Sprenger, J. & Kramer, H. (1928). *Malleus Maleficarum 1484,* translated by Montague Summers, John Rodker, London.

Von Hohenheim, T.B. (Paracelsus) (1565). *Opus Chirurgicum,* National Library of Medicine, Bethesda.

2 An International Perspective — Women in Developing Countries

'Women need to be considered for their own worth, as equal members of society, rather than only as mothers, potential mothers or carers', according to Dr Halfdan Mahler, Director General of the World Health Organization (WHO). It is clear that globally, and particularly in developing countries, women are at a disadvantage in health terms. The social context in which they live means they are less likely to be educated, medicated and even fed. Women have low life expectancy and suffer more from malnutrition and their quality of life and health is affected by repeated childbirth. The lack of adequate contraceptive and reproductive advice and assistance means that reproduction for these women is out of their control. In general, poverty is at the root of these problems within the context of developing countries. Within the health care sector this situation is exemplified where there are fewer opportunities for women in health care provision, other than as carers on an unpaid level, with consequent lesser status.

WOMEN AS CONSUMERS

At present, women's health is measured through morbidity studies, using life expectancy as the indicator. But whilst this may show changes in women's physical well being over time, it tells us nothing about the quality of health during life. According to the United Nations' *Demographic indicators of countries* (1982), projections for 1985, baby girls born at that time would live 13 years longer than those born in 1950. However, there continue to be very large variations below the average, and female babies in poorer countries can still expect to have a shorter life than those in richer countries did 35 years ago (see table 2.1).

Between 1950 and 1985 there were substantial increases in life expectancy in all developing countries as defined by the World Health Organisation. Yet in many of these countries female life expectancy remains unacceptably low. As the *Demographic indicators of countries* (1982) reflect, although developed countries have an average life expectancy of 77 years, 14 of the poorer countries studied in the report, which have a female population of 66 million, have yet to attain a female life expectancy of 50 years; with one exception, these countries are in Sub-Saharan Africa or South Asia.

Table 2.1: 15 Countries with the Lowest Female Life Expectancy, 1980

	Female Life Expectancy years	Total Fertility rate	Infant Mortality rate	Women's Illiteracy rate	GNP per capita US$	Calories % of requirements
World Average (140 countries)	64	3.6	81	34	2,616	107
Afghanistan	41	6.9	205	94	240	75
Chad	42	5.9	143	92	113	76
Ethiopia	43	6.7	143	95	137	74
Gambia	44	6.4	193	88	384	94
Nepal	44	6.2	144	94	135	87
Yemen Arab Rep.	45	6.8	153	98	578	94
Upper Volta	45	6.5	204	95	221	85
Somalia	45	6.1	143	97	283	92
Senegal	45	6.5	141	86	471	95
Niger	45	7.1	140	94	325	94
Mauritania	45	6.9	137	...	414	89
Mali	45	6.7	148	92	196	85
Burundi	45	6.1	117	85	210	92
Angola	45	6.4	148	81	902	90
Bangladesh	47	6.2	133	80	129	85

... not available

(Reprinted with permission from World Priorities, Inc. Washington, D.C., from R.L. Sivard's (1984) *Women ... a world survey*.)

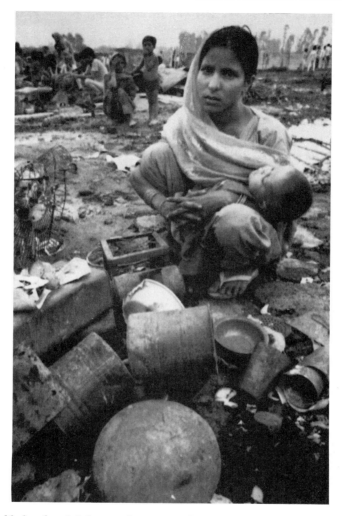

A mother and baby after their home, a hut in an Indian shanty town, was destroyed by fire

According to the United Nation's (1982) 1985 projections, women live four years longer on average than men. However, this differential is far from uniform, and the variations are of interest in illustrating the relationship between women's longevity and the economic-cultural setting (see table 2.1).

The effect of biological differences between women and men, for example oestrogen, often called women's biological advantage, seems to be enhanced in the developed countries. In the US, Japan, and the UK for example, the gap between women's and men's life expectancy appears, according to the United Nations (1982) to have widened in the past 35 years, from 5 years in 1950 to 7 years in 1985. The reasons for this are many and include: decline in cardiovascular diseases among women and sharp increases in mortality from cancer and respiratory disease among men.

Interestingly, there is evidence from the World Bank (1983) of a strong correlation between women's life expectancy and per capita Gross National Product (GNP) in the developed countries. While benefiting from medical and other advantages associated with socio-economic progress, women seem to have been less inclined to adopt some of the unhealthy habits often associated with affluence: cigarette smoking, excessive consumption of food and alcohol, fast driving (and high accident rates) and high levels of stress. However, this advantage may lessen over time due to changes in women's life styles. The recent increases in women's smoking habits and the increased stress as women deal with the competing demands of the home and the workplace may mean that women start to emulate men in their disease patterns, although all of this is highly speculative without the benefit of research findings.

The United Nations' *Demographic indicators of countries* (1982) reflects a narrowing of sex differences in life expectancy in the developing countries. The Third World average in 1985 was 62 years for women and 60 years for men. In India, Nepal and Pakistan, the difference in life expectancy is actually in men's favour, with men living on average a year longer.

Female advantage in life expectancy at birth is a nearly universal phenomenon. Yet there are vulnerable ages in which females are more at risk of dying than males in Third World countries. These periods occur during early childhood and the childbearing ages.

In Asia and Africa, higher female mortality in both these periods of life appears to be associated with the relatively low cultural position accorded girls and women. This holds particularly true in rural areas, where boys are much more highly valued than girls. Because of their greater economic potential, boys are given correspondingly greater care. Sivard (1984) reports that allocation of food in developing countries, from where data is gathered, is 16 per cent higher for boys under five than girls. Infant malnutrition runs at 14 per cent for girls and 5 per cent for boys. Access to health care for female children is also limited. The delay in seeking medical treatment for male children is 23 per cent of all children who eventually receive treatment, whereas for female children it is 44 per cent.

In India and Bangladesh, for example, female mortality between 1 and 5 years of age may range as high as 30–50 per cent above male mortality (Sivard 1984). Boys are given more medical attention and more food. There is also anecdotal evidence of infanticide of girl babies in China and continuing widow burning in the Indian subcontinent. In 1979 the Chinese government introduced its controversial one child per family program, in an attempt to limit population growth. The United Nations' *Demographic yearbook* (1984) estimates the number of baby girls to have been killed since 1979 at 250 000.

It is difficult to ascertain accurate data on world wide maternal mortality. Less than half the member states of WHO measure maternal mortality and nearly two-thirds of developing countries cannot measure maternal mortality. In the countries where it is measured the major causes are anaemia due to malnutrition and infection. The United Nations *Demographic yearbook* (1984) reported that in Latin America half the maternal mortality figures are due to illegal abortion.

CONTRIBUTING FACTORS

Unemployment, low pay, and unskilled work increase impoverishment among women. Throughout the world, there are more women than men who are poor, and their numbers are growing. In the US, one of the most prosperous countries on earth, Sivard (1984) reports that two out of every three adults living below the poverty level in 1983 were women; one elderly woman in six was poor; one in every two poor families was headed by a woman.

In Third World countries where traditional societies are breaking down as men migrate to seek work, fight wars or desert their impoverished families, the poverty of women is accentuated. According to Sivard (1984) those households with female heads form a large majority of the poorest and sickest families.

Malnutrition

The factors affecting women's health contribute not only to the broad differences in women's life expectancy but also to differential morbidity. There are two areas, where it is possible to obtain practical information, which offer some explanation about illness in women in developing countries.

The first of these areas is malnutrition. One-quarter of the population in developing countries is undernourished, but precisely what proportion of these people are women is not known. Although women are not alone in suffering from

---

Public health in the Third World — The Pacific

The Republic of Vanuatu lies 2000 km off the north-east coast of Australia in the Pacific Ocean. It is an archipelago of 80 or more islands. It stretches 900 km from north to south, and has a population of 138 000. It has a tropical climate, with a wet season from November to May and a dry one from June to October. Of the population, 97% are Melanesian and 45% are aged 15 years or younger. Most of the population live in small villages. There are only two major towns: Port Vila, the capital, with 15 000 inhabitants on Efate Island; and Luganville on Espiritu Santo. The gross national product is about US$300 per inhabitant.

The issue of women's health is not one the country has faced directly, but the public health campaigns to control malaria, leprosy, and tuberculosis obviously benefit all the population. All these diseases are major problems. Malaria and tuberculosis are endemic. As well, The National Health Service has an expanded immunisation program, a nutrition education campaign, and also a primary health care program which not only assists in the national program of immunisation begun in 1982 but also provides help with the water supply. This is inadequate in many areas — up to 90% of households lack water on some islands. Only 20% of households have toilets, but almost all villages have public facilities.

An average of 80% of pregnant women (ranging from 45% to 95% of pregnant women depending on the island of residence) are examined by a doctor at least once during pregnancy. Approximately 70% of the estimated 15 380 annual births are attended by a doctor. However, the infant mortality rate is relatively high; it is estimated at between 6% to 10.3%.

The life expectancy for men is 61 years, and 59 years for women.

It can be seen that any improvement in public health will be of benefit to women as well. Issues of specific concern to women in Australian society are perhaps not well appreciated in Vanuatu.

Adapted from Patrick Bastien, *The medical journal of Australia*, 1990, 1, 13–17.

malnutrition, social custom often dictates that malnutrition occurs in greater numbers among women and girls. Royston (1982) reports that women are often subject to food taboos and in many societies it is customary for the men to eat first, boys next, girls and women last. In times of shortage, protein goes to the men.

Malnutrition, measured by nutritional anaemia, is considered by WHO as the most significant health problem for Third World women. According to Royston (1982), close to half of all the women of child-bearing age (15–49 years) and 60 per cent of pregnant women are malnourished. Compare this with 4 to 7 per cent of women in European countries and 6 per cent in the US (see figure 2.1).

Although not normally fatal, anaemia, which may also be a consequence of iron-deficiency related to frequent childbearing, lowers resistance, limits the capacity for physically demanding work and seriously erodes the quality of life. Malnutrition and iron deficiency anaemia become a vicious cycle, affecting both the pregnant woman's health and that of her unborn child.

Figure 2.1: Prevalence of nutritional anaemia among women 15–49 years, population 1975

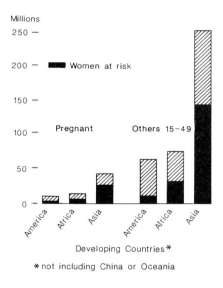

(Reprinted with permission from World Priorities, Inc. Washington, D.C., from R.L. Sivard's (1984) *Women ... a world survey*)

Childbirth

The other factor affecting women's health in developing countries is childbearing. Repeated childbirth, short intervals between births and pregnancy at an early age all pose high risks to women's health. The United Nations reports in its *Infant mortality: world estimates and projections 1950–2025* (1983) that although world populations are decreasing, on average 3.8 children are born to a woman in developing countries (compared with 2.0 in developed) and, in some countries, national averages are still as high as 7.9 children. It is estimated that at any one time, one woman in six in the age group from 15–49 years is pregnant in developing countries (excluding China), compared with one woman in seventeen in developed countries.

In some countries, infant mortality runs as high as 20 per cent — one birth in five. According to the United Nations (1983), in India, if a woman has six surviving children over one year of age, then in the course of her 30 year reproductive life span she has been pregnant eight times. Given that each liveborn infant is generally breastfed for 2–3 years, then the mother will have spent 200 months, or 50 to 60 per cent of her reproductive years, in pregnancy and breastfeeding.

Every pregnancy places great strains on the health status of the mother. The United Nations Food and Agricultural Organisation's *Monthly bulletin of statistics* (1985) estimates that about 418 550 kilojoules are expended per pregnancy and about 7534 kilojoules per day during breastfeeding. Women are often too impoverished to adjust their diet to meet these demands. For this reason, malnutrition increases maternal mortality and overall mortality during women's fundamentally strong mid-life years.

Because the number of deaths resulting from childbirth are seriously underreported in the Third World, it is difficult to judge the full extent of women's maternal mortality. However, according to WHO estimates (UN *Demographic yearbook* (1984)), maternal causes are among the five leading causes of death in the 15–44 years age group; in one-third of the countries maternal causes come first or second in overall death rates. Sivard's (1984) studies indicate that in developing countries, complications of pregnancy and delivery may account for one-quarter of the deaths among women in the 15–49 years age group (see figures 2.2 and 2.3).

Figure 2. 2: Life expectancy of women at birth   **Figure 2.3:** Maternal mortality

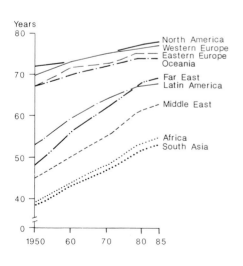

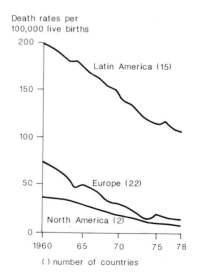

(Reprinted with permission from World Priorities, Inc. Washington, D.C., from R.L. Sivard's (1984) *Women ... a world survey*)

Family planning

Family planning programs are one factor which can make an appreciable difference in the survival rates of women and infants. Family planning makes it possible for women to avoid high risk pregnancies and the illegal abortions which are a major cause of death among women in many developing countries.

Family Planning, the World Bank (1983) notes, also has a wide range of positive benefits for women. By enabling them to control their fertility, it enlarges the choices open to them, freeing them to become better educated, to improve opportunities for their children and to increase their own participation in economic development. The Bank reports that 85 countries in the Third World, representing about 95 per cent of its population, now provide some form of public support for family planning programs. Yet use of contraception varies widely among regions and countries and also between urban and rural areas. In Africa, where infant and maternal mortality are highest, poverty is most extreme, and population growth most rapid, contraceptive use is the lowest. In virtually all developing countries surveyed, the majority (50 to 90 per cent) of married women of childbearing age want either to limit or space births. Many publicly supported programs do not provide adequate coverage, however, and there is a substantial unmet need for user-oriented family planning services which also offer general health-care counselling for women, particularly in rural areas.

Education and literacy

UNESCO (1982) reports that discrimination in educational opportunities for girls and women is world wide. It contributes to the lower socio-economic status of women and therefore their poverty and illness. Unfortunately, the increase in girls' enrolment since 1950 has so far failed to eliminate a broad disparity between the sexes. At all levels of education, boys still represent a majority of students. According to world enrolment totals, at both the primary and secondary levels, 55 per cent of students are boys, and 45 per cent are girls; at the third level, the ratio changes slightly to 57 per cent boys, 43 per cent girls (see figures 2.4, 2.5).

Behind these averages are continuing major differences in national and regional patterns. Developing countries in general reveal greater sex inequalities in education than do developed. According to the US National Center of Educational Statistics (1984) approximately 28 per cent of all girls aged between 12 and 17 attend school in developing countries compared with 85 per cent in developed countries. At successively higher educational levels the inequality becomes more pronounced. At the university level in the Third World men outnumber women almost two to one.

Low literacy rates for women as well as broad sex differentials have a common denominator in poverty. At least 60 per cent of the 500 million women who are unable to read and write live in countries where the average per capita income in 1980 was below US$300 (US National Center of Educational Statistics 1984).

Sivard's (1984) statistics show that in trend and geographic comparisons, there has been a record increase in the number of literate women in the world, a gain of close to 500 million since 1960 to over one billion currently. Literacy has outstripped the rise in adult population as well, so that the literacy rate for women

Figure 2.4: Girls' enrolment in school and school-age population

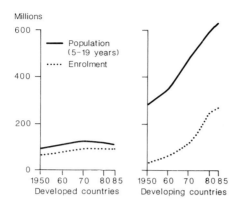

(Reprinted with permission from World Priorities, Inc. Washington, D.C., from R.L. Sivard's (1984) *Women ... a world survey*)

Figure 2.5: Enrolment of girls and boys, first and second levels of education

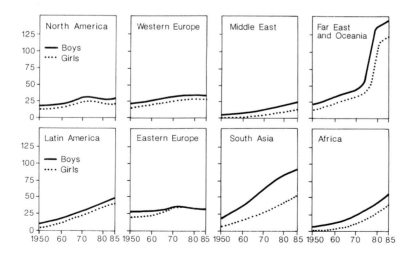

(Reprinted with permission from World Priorities, Inc. Washington, D.C., from R.L. Sivard's (1984) *Women ... a world survey*)

(not including China) is now 68 per cent, as compared with 59 per cent in 1960. In developing countries however, literacy rates for girls are less than 33 per cent whereas for boys they are over 50 per cent.

The wide gap in literacy rates between men and women has not diminished significantly with the years. According to UNESCO, the estimated global differential in 1985 amounts to 10 percentage points, i.e. 78 per cent of adult men are able to read and write compared with 68 per cent of adult women, a discrepancy which means that in the world (excluding China) there are 130 million more women than men who are illiterate. In developed countries there is virtually no gap between the sexes, but in the Third World a literacy average of 50 per cent contrasts with 68 per cent for men.

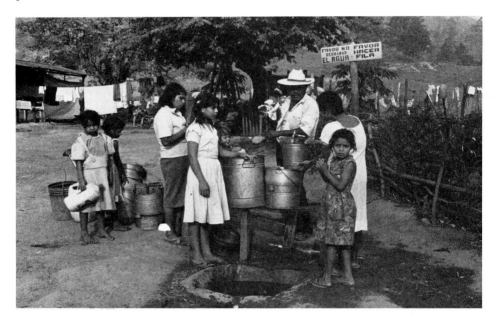

The non-paid health care work of women includes the supply of clean water

WOMEN AS PROVIDERS

The following observations about women as health care providers were made in WHO's (1985) *Multinational study on women as providers of health care*: the workforce tends to be predominantly female; epitomises the functions viewed traditionally as female, e.g. caring, consoling, counselling, cooking, cleaning and educating; and mirrors imbalance in society with women playing subordinate roles.

Bui Dang Ha Doan (1981) found that the rate of participation in the health labour force of women was much higher than in the total labour force. In developing countries this trend was more pronounced. For example, in the Dominican Republic, the ratio is five times as great and in Iraq it is 13 times as great. WHO

The global epidemiological pattern

Since the first cases of AIDS were described in June 1981, Governments around the world have approached the epidemic by grossly underestimating its potential impact as a major international public health problem. The AIDS Program of the World Health Organization estimates that there are more than 250 000 cases of AIDS and that between five and ten million people are infected with the HIV. Because the disease process is slow, taking many years before illness occurs, the overall caseload is expected to get much worse during the next decade. Surveillance of case incidence is estimated to be 80% to 90% accurate in developed countries, but less than 50% in developing countries where under-reporting, under-recognition and under-diagnosis contribute to this situation.

Africa

The pattern of AIDS in Africa is distinct from that observed in Western countries, but is similar to Central American countries like Haiti. In Africa, the AIDS pandemic is focused in Central, Eastern and Southern African urban areas where cases primarily exist in heterosexual men and women. The ration of male to female cases is about one. The World Health Organization currently estimates that the 100 000 cases of AIDS now occurring will reach 400 000 by the mid-1990s. The long term impact of the epidemic is difficult to predict, but given that 10% to 25% of reproductive age women are infected in some urban areas, the early childhood mortality is expected to significantly increase within 5 years. In addition, the total adult mortality from AIDS will place tremendous strain on the health-care systems of those countries least able to cope with the burden. Fortunately the HIV is found predominantly in urban areas where only 10% to 20% of people live. If this pattern changes through increasing rural-urban migration, the epidemic situation may become even more uncontrollable.

Americas

The epidemiological pattern of HIV in the American continent is generally similar to that of most industrialised countries of Europe and Oceania. The first cases of AIDS were reported amongst homosexual and bisexual men who still remain the group at highest risk of infection. Intravenous drug users are becoming an increasingly important risk group. The male to female ration of AIDS cases is about ten to one to fifteen to one. Blood product recipients were an early risk group, but this was prevented by a widespread blood screening program introduced in 1985. The future of the epidemic on this continent is no more optimistic than it is in Africa. Medical services are more developed in North America where the overall annual cost is estimated to approach $15 billion by 1992. In South America, the epidemic is expected to spread more rapidly into the general heterosexual community because sexual promiscuity with female prostitutes is widely practised by males. Health care in these countries is generally of a low standard, which may facilitate transmission of HIV because untreated intercurrent infections predispose to viral infection.

Europe

In Europe the epidemiology of AIDS varies from area to area. Western Europe shows a similar pattern to the United States where homosexual and bisexual males and intravenous drug users comprise more than 90% of cases. Northern Europe has mainly homosexually acquired cases, while Spain and Italy have mainly cases acquired via sharing contaminated syringes. Eastern European countries have recently started to report cases to WHO. Their infections have usually been acquired in Western countries, via homosexual activity or drug use. Very few indigenously acquired infections have been reported, indicating that different social behaviours regarding sexual contact and drug use may delay the epidemic in these countries.

Asia

In Asia there are just over 200 reported cases. This indicates the relatively recent spread of HIV into this region. No single Asian country has a high prevalence of AIDS, with most infections acquired through sexual contact with visitors from epidemic countries. Recent data from Thailand indicates that the situation necessary for rapid spread of HIV may have already arrived. Researchers in Bangkok have documented an increase in the infection rate amongst intravenous drug users from zero per cent in 1986 to one per cent in 1987 to sixteen per cent in early 1988. It is estimated that there are 60 000 drug users of whom 10 000 may already be infected. As many practise prostitution with foreign tourists, the risk to other Asian countries will become more important over time.

Julian Gold, Bruce White, Andrew Morlet and David Cooper (1989). Epidemiology of Human Immunodeficiency Virus Infection, in R. Richmond and D. Wakefield (eds) *AIDS and other sexually transmitted diseases*, W.B. Saunders, Sydney.

(1985) suggests that women constituted approximately 95 per cent of the world's nurses, 39 per cent of physicians, 33 per cent of pharmacists, and 15 per cent of dentists. Information about career status, income and decision making roles is fragmented. It is available from some developed countries where the opportunities for women in the health professions are poor.

In both developed and developing countries women's roles in non-formal health systems is acknowledged to be much greater. Data compiled from a range of ILO *Yearbook of labour statistics* reports that in developing countries the non-paid health care work of women includes the supply of clean water (women are the main haulers of water for domestic consumption), and ensuring sanitary conditions and producing edible food (African women spend about 13 hours pounding enough maize to feed their families for 4 days).

Whilst women in developing countries are primarily concerned with daily survival and have little time to organise concerted campaigns to improve access to and quality of health care services, two types of activities are prevalent amongst these countries: large centralised women's health groups, e.g. Maendeleo Ya Wanawake and the Breastfeeding Information Group, both in Nairobi; and village level initiatives for rural women, e.g. The Rural Women's Health Group in South India.

Some women believe the development of self help groups is inadvertently helping to postpone much needed reforms. Once again the more formal structures of health care are incorporating women's unpaid work. Women are conducting unpaid work in health care whilst governments pretend that they are discharging their responsibilities. WHO's Regional Committee for Europe (1981) notes that the promotion of self care is likely to increase women's workload and widen the socio-economic gap which promotes women's illness. Women's input, albeit unpaid, is important structurally. The view of women as consumers has now achieved some status through the self-help movement, e.g. Boston Women's Health Collective were integral in the early days of the women's health movement.

CASE STUDY

It had been raining heavily, so there were puddles in the potholes on the dirt road. The sun was glinting in them, and the children were chasing one another — and the dogs — in and out of them, laughing and shouting as they did so. Julia unlocked the door of the Community Health Centre, and showed May in. None of the others had arrived yet, so she had time to show her supervisor the new child health cards which had arrived. May is the Regional Nursing Advisor for Community Health, and Julia is the nurse responsible for the Health Centre, which takes care of the health needs for four villages. May had always felt a glow of pride as she walked into this clinic, and especially today it looked light and welcoming with the late afternoon sun pouring through the windows. May and Julia had initiated the idea of this Centre, and many hours of effort had preceded its opening almost a year ago.

More barking and shouting outside heralded the arrival of the three village women who are the community representatives and coordinators for the Centre. Julia hurried out, and while greeting them, ordered her own children and their friends to walk back home to the other end of the village.

Soon the five women were sitting around a table in Julia's office discussing the topic which had brought May out to the Centre. In three weeks time it will have been opened a year, and the Minister of Health wants to bring some officials from other regions to show them what such a Centre can achieve. He wants them to present some of the achievements of their new services, which he must have heard about after May submitted her latest report to the Health Department.

Julia showed the others a new set of figures which she has prepared for this meeting.

'This information shows that the mothers' management of diarrhoea in babies is improving. If you look at this chart you can see that the number of admissions to the clinic has been increasing steadily as the months have passed. During the last three months the admissions were 100 per cent higher than in the first three months. At first we were worried that this showed that there was increasing diarrhoea among the babies, and couldn't understand why there were a percentage who seemed to be more sick than we had seen before. The answer came from those books you sent May — there are a greater number of sick children, but that is because there are fewer dying. So, in the last six months four times as many mothers gave their babies oral rehydration therapy properly, compared to our first six months. Nearly all of these women had been to our education groups, and the ones who hadn't had read material given to them by the ones who came. The death rate is down by something like 30 per cent in the past two months, compared to the first two months of the Centre's operation.'

'There is still a lot of work to do though, because for some it was too late by the time they came to us; and there is some confusion about how to give the solution. Yet, there are dozens of children running and playing out there, because we have given them the opportunity to live. That's pretty exciting, isn't it?' There was no disagreement, they all felt proud to hear those results.

After some discussion they decided to also present the way in which they are making new targets for the next year. Two targets are to increase the spacing of pregnancies, and to increase the percentage of children immunised.

May is pleased with this suggestion, because it is an area in which there seems a lot of confusion among the health workers she supervises. 'We can document the process we go through over the next few weeks — deciding on our exact objectives, which women we wish to work with especially ... how we want to improve our service ... and of course evaluating whether that has an impact or not. And then ... I could use it again in other villages, and share it with other regional supervisors.' She sounds very enthusiastic, and laughs with the others at how clever they are.

Almost everything seems settled. May brings up one last point before they close the meeting. 'By the way, there will be someone from the Department of Health coming, because they want the Minister to announce the building of a new well, and tap water supply on the far south side of the village. I hadn't heard about it before, but I guess... she did not get to finish her sentence. Vinnie, the community coordinator exclaims 'A new well on the far south side?! May, are you serious? Yes, I see by your face you are.'

One of the other women breaks in 'May, we have been through this battle before. The affluent farmers in that area want the water supply to improve their crop growing. It's not going to help women or children one scrap. In fact it will delay getting water taps to the areas in the villages where we desperately need them for household water.'

Vinnie spoke again 'The farmers have been lobbying for this, and we have been fighting for water taps so women will not have to spend so many hours carrying water to their homes. We have to start attacking again. They have got to the administrators and politicians with their smooth economic arguments!' She turns to May, who is thinking that she has been rather naive for not questioning the department about this more closely. 'You see, you really need us, or you would be part of the exploitation of women, while you thought you were doing a good job...'

REFERENCES

Bui Dang Ha Doan (1981). The participation of women in the health care system: an international panorama, in World Health Organisation, (1985), *Multinational study on women as providers of health care*, WHO, Geneva.

International Labour Organisation, *Yearbook of Labour Statistics*, International Labour Organisation, Geneva.

Royston, E. (1982). The prevalence of nutritional anaemia in women in developing countries, *WHO Statistical Quarterly* No. 2.

Sivard, R.L. (1984). *Women ... a world survey*, World Priorities, Washington D.C.

UNESCO (1982). *Trends and projections of enrolment by level of education and by age 1960–2000*, Statistical Yearbook, UNESCO.

United Nations (1983). Infant mortality: world estimates and projections, 1950–2025, *United Nations Population Bulletin*, No. 13.

United Nations (1984). *United nations demographic yearbook*, Pan American Health Organization, Washington DC.

United Nations Food and Agricultural Organization (1985). *Monthly bulletin of statistics*, United Nations, Rome.

United Nations Population Division (1982). *Demographic indicators of countries*, United Nations, New York.

US National Center of Educational Statistics (1984). *Digest of education statistics*, US National Center of Education Statistics, Washington D.C.

World Bank (1983). *Per capita GNP figures, world military and social expenditures*, World Bank, Geneva.

World Health Organisation (1985). *Multinational study on women as providers of health care*, WHO, Geneva.

World Health Organisation, Regional Committee for Europe, (1981). *Regional strategy for attaining health for all by the year 2000: progress report*, WHO, Copenhagen.

3 Women's Major Health Needs

This chapter aims to provide an overview of what is known about the priorities for women's health. The major focus will be on describing the health needs of women and evaluating the adequacy of existing information sources. The need for intervention programs will be identified where possible, although there is currently often too little information about potential interventions to propose priorities in a systematic manner.

WHAT ARE THE MAJOR HEALTH NEEDS OF WOMEN?

Identification of those problems which have the greatest burden of illness for women is critical, if the overall health of women in the community is to be improved. An understanding of the major health problems provides direction for agencies supplying services to women, helps identify the skills needed by health care providers and indicates the needs for further research and program development. Determining the major health needs can also provide an agenda for action, by enabling the setting of future goals and targets. The most effective type of needs assessment combines information from a wide variety of sources, including mortality and morbidity data, perceptions of health needs among health care providers and women themselves, as well as demographic and preventive health information (see Table 3.1).

31

When the major health problems have been established, it will be necessary to describe and evaluate interventions to reduce their occurrence. The programs to be implemented must ultimately be determined based on their ability to reduce the burden of illness in a cost effective manner. Currently, there is very little information about the relative effectiveness of many of the intervention strategies which are proposed or implemented for women's health.

Table 3.1: Information sources for assessing health needs

Health status indicators

e.g.   mortality
        morbidity

Opinion-based information sources

e.g.   community perceptions
        lobby groups
        health care providers

Underlying factors

e.g.   health risk behaviours
        socio-economic and role profiles
        adequacy of health care

HEALTH STATUS INDICATORS

The first type of information about health needs comes from information collected about the extent of and causes of death and illness, known as health status indicators.

Mortality

In Australia in 1987, the life expectancy for females was 79.5 years compared with 73.01 years for males (Australian Bureau of Statistics 1988). Females of all ages have a lower death rate than do males. However the difference is most marked in the age group 15 to 24 where the rate for females is much less than that of males (Australian Bureau of Statistics 1988).

During this century Australian women have always had a greater life expectancy than men. In the period, 1901–1911, for example, the life expectancy for males was 55.2 years and for females 58.8 years (Australian Bureau of Statistics 1984). However, the differences in life expectancy between men and women have increased throughout this century, with women living increasingly longer relative to men. Figure 3.1 shows data from the USA illustrating these trends. During this century the health care system has been more effective in dealing with the health problems which primarily affect women (e.g. childbirth, cancer of the cervix).

Figure 3.1: Sex mortality ratio (male/female) by age, United States, 1900–1980. Based on mortality rates.

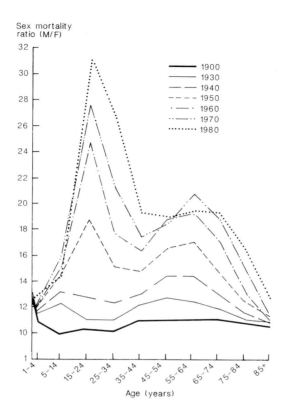

(Wingard 1984)

Despite the differences in life expectancy, there is a striking similarity between the common causes of death for women and men in all age groups. In younger age groups, the main causes of death for both men and women are road traffic and other accidents, while in later life, heart disease, cerebrovascular disease and stroke and cancer are the major killers. Figure 3.2 shows the relative gain in life expectancy for men and women if specific causes of death were to be eliminated.

Common types of cancer in women include bowel, breast and lung cancers. Although little can be done to reduce the prevalence of bowel cancer, smoking cessation will limit the incidence of lung cancer. Lung cancer is of particular concern for women, since rates of smoking are increasing among young women and it is therefore expected that we will see a higher rate of lung cancer among women in the near future. Mammography screening has been shown to significantly decrease mortality from breast cancer (Tabar et al. 1989); the implementation of community wide mammography screening programs should be among the priorities for women's health. However, there is some argument about this. It is possible that mammography increases risk for low-risk groups. It has been suggested that selective screening may reduce mortality better than universal screening. Ensuring

Figure 3.2: Gain in life expectancy at age one year if specific causes of death were to be eliminated.

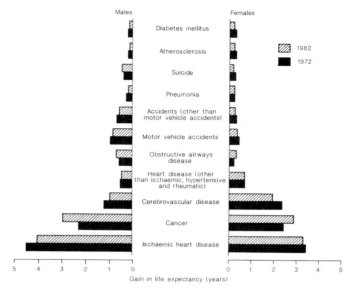

(Australian Bureau of Statistics 1983)

adequate screening for cervical cancer has also been perceived as a major health need for women. Although cervical cancer is not common, the majority of deaths from this disease are preventable through screening programs using the Papanicolau smear. However, currently as few as 18 per cent of women may have annual screens (Mitchell and Medley 1987).

Morbidity

While good measures of mortality exist, there are fewer adequate methods of assessing morbidity. It is sometimes argued that one of the ways in which the existing health care system discriminates against women is in its focus on mortality: women's major health needs lie in improving morbidity rather than mortality. However our health care system continues to focus predominantly on mortality rather than morbidity.

Information about community morbidity comes from several sources. Community surveys using direct measures of diseases such as hypertension or psychological disturbance have been undertaken, most usually directed at a specific disease. Rates of referrals to specialists, drug prescriptions, cancer or other registers all provide some measure of the morbidity in a community. However, most of these sources tend to provide information about the occurrence of specific diseases rather than allowing comparisons between different diseases. Accordingly, health care utilisation rates and community surveys of self-reported morbidity have been used most frequently to explore the health needs of groups such as women since they can provide information about a wide variety of disease types.

Measurement of health care utilisation

Health care utilisation data show consistently higher rates of health care use among women than men. In NSW in 1986, the number of hospital admissions for males was 180 per 1000 and for females 235 (Australian Bureau of Statistics 1990). In NSW in 1981, women stayed longer in hospital, with an average 22.3 bed days, excluding those for pregnancy, compared with 16.9 for males (Australian Bureau of Statistics 1984). Women are also more frequent utilisers of general practice. In the *Newcastle Primary Care Study* (Dickinson et al. 1989) 61 per cent of the 2300 general practice patients attending 56 general practitioners were female. Similarly, the Australian Bureau of Statistics reported an average of 14.4 consultations per 1000 women and 8.1 per 1000 men in a two week period (Australian Bureau of Statistics 1983). Figure 3.3 shows the number of people attending their doctor for different reasons as assessed by the ABS study.

In assessing health care utilisation data, it is also important to consider the role 'iatrogenic' illness has in increasing usage rates. Since young women attend doctors more frequently than men, for problems such as contraception and pre and post natal care, it is argued that the chances of being diagnosed as suffering from another health problem increase. The National Heart Foundation's 1983 *Risk Factor Prevalence Study* indicates that men with hypertension are less likely to be treated than women. In part, this may be because women are more likely to visit the doctor and to have their hypertension diagnosed. The diagnosis of hypertension will then lead to more consultations in the future.

Research exploring whether women are more or less willing than men to seek help when they are ill has yielded mixed findings with some studies showing women more likely to seek help and others finding no gender differences. In a recent review of this literature, Waldron (1983) concluded that for a given level of

Figure 3.3: Number of persons who consulted a doctor in the three months before interview by the main reason for most recent consultation (a).

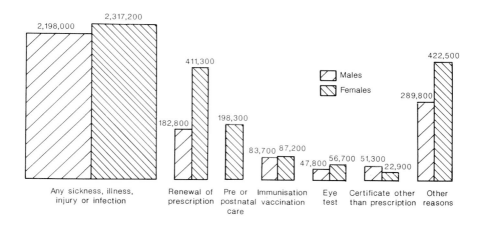

(Australian Bureau of Statistics 1983)

self perceived health, women may be more likely than men to make a doctor visit for less serious illness and preventive care, but not for life threatening illness or those that interfere with normal activities such as myocardial infarctions or cancer. Table 3.2 shows the number of women per 1000 visiting their doctor in the past two weeks for each of the listed health problems, as reported in the *Australian Health Survey* 1983.

Table 3.2

Illness	Women	Male:Female ratio
Endocrine	41	0.77
Mental disorders	60	0.59
Nervous systems and sense organs	138	0.77
Circulatory system	199	0.60
Respiratory system	313	0.89
Digestive system	83	0.92
Genito urinary system	98	0.23
Skin and subcutaneous tissue	88	0.83
Muscoskeletal	161	0.95
Other, specified	161	1.17
Symptoms and ill-defined conditions	98	0.74
Other reasons		
Check-up	86	0.69
Pregnancy	96	-
Immunisation	22	0.77

(Based on Australian Bureau of Statistics 1983)

Self-reported morbidity

The second source of information about morbidity comes from community surveys of self-reported morbidity. According to the *Australian Health Survey* (1983) women were more likely to report days of reduced activity than men. Women reported spending more days in bed due to illness, with 528 days reported by women and 393 days by men.

Forty-eight per cent of women reported one or more chronic conditions and 43 per cent of men reported having one or more chronic conditions (Australian Bureau of Statistics 1977). A similar pattern is evident in the reporting of recent illness. In the 1983 survey, 572 men and 673 women per 1000 in the population reported at least one illness condition in the preceding 2 weeks. The greatest differences in the frequency with which specific conditions were reported by men and women was, not surprisingly, in the genito-urinary system — over 7 times greater for women. Other conditions with a large difference in reporting rates between women and men included: mental disorders (nearly twice); problems with the circulatory system and nervous system disorders.

The most commonly reported illness conditions among women relate to four main categories and some miscellaneous problems as shown in Table 3.3. Problems most often reported were related to headaches, nerves and insomnia. The rates of these problems were very high particularly for non-specific headaches. Infections of the upper respiratory tract were also common with women reporting a high prevalence of colds and influenza. Skeletal and cardiovascular problems were also common, as were menstrual problems.

Table 3.3: most commonly reported causes of illness episodes by women

Self-reported illness episodes	
Number of women who experienced illness conditions in previous 2 weeks ('000)	
Nervous problems	
Headaches from trivial causes	923
Stress headaches	353
Migraine	172
Nerves and tension	337
Insomnia	271
Respiratory tract infections	
Acute nasopharyngitis	496
Influenza	247
Sinusitis	153
Cough/sore throat	194
Skeletal problems	
Arthritis	370
Back problems	168
Injuries	235
Cardiovascular	
Hypertension	653
Heart disease	210
Miscellaneous	
Menstrual problems	247
Constipation	219
Eczema	294
Dental problems	350

(Based on Australian Bureau of Statistics 1983)

However, some care should be taken in interpreting information from self report surveys of illness. Self reports can be made inaccurate by difficulties in recalling illness episodes. Women may be more likely to report illness than men because social stereotyping makes illness more acceptable in women. Women's greater knowledge about health and concern with family health has also been argued to make women more aware of illness and thus more likely to report its occurrence.

Community Policing Squad in Victoria

It's 4pm and the first hour of the shift has passed waiting in vain for a woman who rang to say she needed accommodation, drinking tea and studying the case book. Sergeant Trish Duke decides it's time to head off around the city and inner suburban beat [with] Constable Jason Halls — a trainee doing his mandatory two weeks with a CPS unit. This is his last day.

First stop is a welfare check on an 80-year-old Italian who speaks no English and lives alone. Duke has been calling on her regularly since hearing eight months ago that the woman wasn't well and had a few problems. As usual, she is sitting at the window watching passers-by. 'Thank you very much' is her only English — repeated constantly as Duke checks the kitchen, the woman's tablets and general comfort.

Next stop is another welfare check — on a young mother in a Housing Commission flat, reported not to be coping with her two children. Budgeting and alcohol abuse play a major role in such cases, says Duke, who has been 18 months with CPS and 13 years on the force.

'Mostly, it's not as bad as people say. Sometimes, families can't cope and want you to help but are too frightened to ring themselves or don't know who to ask. They're often glad we come in because they want the pressure taken off them for a while.'

Other than in cases of obvious child abuse or neglect where they would issue a protection application, the CPS connects families with local welfare agencies and follows up with regular checks. After today's visit, the children wave us off from the balcony and we leave in a blaze of blue flashing light — on request. This is a big turnaround, says Duke. 'Last time, we were abused and called for a back-up unit but a lot has happened since and there's no alcohol present now.'

The car radio directs us to a regular police job, attending the site of a break-in and attempted car theft. It's 6pm and the radio is running hot with calls to post-football pub brawls. We are called as back-up to a domestic violence incident. On goes the blue light as we dash through red lights, only to be told a minute from the scene that we are not needed. So it's back into the city for a take-away dinner, driving straight down the pedestrian mall to park outside a pizza parlour. The 15-minute wait is taken up searching through seedy fun parlours looking for a 14-year-old girl who has broken a couple of court orders.

Back at Russell Street, we meet 'Tony', an undersized 12-year-old with blonde-tipped hair and a ferocious expression, leaning on the squad room table head in hands and refusing to answer questions. Constable Karen Nicks and Brad Mason, the other CPS team rostered on tonight, have collected him from the Collingwood police after he was found wandering drunk with a gang. He hasn't been home since the previous night and has been staying with street kids in a Fitzroy squat. They've told him that the police bash kids; hence the hostility and refusal to give his correct name and address until told of the possible consequences — a protection application weekend in a boys' home and a Children's Court appearance on Monday.

Duke goes to work on Tony while Nicks works the telephone trying to find his father — who isn't home, doesn't have the phone on and hasn't reported the boy missing.

Slowly, Duke learns that Tony was sent to his father three weeks ago — from Sydney — by his mother, who has other children and wants to remarry.

'Do you realise how important it is to find your Dad?' she insists, then touches the heart ... 'What happened with you and Dad?'

Unexpectedly, Tony bursts into tears — a tired, frightened little boy. But still he can't or won't remember names, addresses, telephone numbers. By now, Nicks is tracing him as a missing person in NSW.

'Don't worry, we're not going to charge you; we're only trying to get you home, so we must find your Dad,' says Duke. Nothing.

'Do you know what happens to little boys on the streets?'

Yes, says Tony, they get raped. Does he know what that means? No. So Duke spells it out. Tony's only refrain by now is that he wants to go home, yet all he knows of Dad is that he's a part-owner of a restaurant which Nicks is unable to trace. Just as we are about to leave and search for it, the phone rings. It's Tony's Dad, who has been driving around searching for the boy. The father is on his way in.

Back on the road at 8.30pm, we check on a couple of old ladies frightened by obscene phone calls. Then we're scratching gravel again for the dash to where vandals are smashing a suburban railway station. Broken glass is everywhere, boys scattering up the tracks in both directions. The mostly young crowd at the station has been harassed for money. Some of the girls are crying. Only one youth volunteers information. The transit police arrive and we leave to attend a child custody situation at risk of flaring up.

Three-year-old Holly was supposed to be returned at 6pm from an access visit to her father and grandmother. At 8pm, mother Tania rang the local police who asked us to accompany her to the grandmother's house. The child has an ear infection and there's a doctor's certificate saying she should not be moved that night. Duke tries to talk Tania out of doing so but she won't budge. Holly is taken out of bed, dressed and carried to the car by Halls.

On the way to check out Tony's squat of the previous night, a rare police-in-trouble call comes over the radio. We speed to the scene of nearby domestic violence, only to find every other patrol car already there. A policeman is taken to hospital with a fractured hand. We raid the squat with a back-up unit, hoping to find a missing teenager. But, despite evidence of habitation, no-one is there.

By 11.10pm, we are back at Russell Street. Tony and Dad have gone after Nicks spent the remainder of her shift talking through their problems. Tony has only seen his father twice in eight years, so there have been discipline problems.

'But the father wants to try and I felt a protection order was the wrong way to go at this time — it would devastate him,' says Nicks, a social welfare worker before joining the force.

She has arranged support from a local social worker and spent time with Tony explaining that he has a chance with his father at which they both have to work.

No, they don't take all this home — except for early on — says Duke, recalling a distressed trainee recently who took a child from its mother in stressful circumstances, changed and fed it at the station and later in the shift was called to attend a cot death.

Jan McGuiness, *The Bulletin*, 8 May 1990

Waldron (1983) reviewed 12 studies comparing self-reported morbidity with physician ratings. She concluded that when compared with physician ratings, women are more likely to judge themselves as in poor general health than men.

Another problem with self report morbidity surveys is that the measures of morbidity are not very sensitive. The use of measures such as bed days or illness episodes appears to equate minor health problems such as hayfever with severe problems such as heart attacks. The conditions of women's lives are very different to those of men: women are more likely to be at home taking care of small children or elderly relatives. An illness which results in a bed day for a mother of two pre-schoolers is likely to be more severe than for someone involved in full time paid employment.

Opinion based information

The third type of information that is useful in assessing the health needs of women is the perceptions of different groups about health needs. Perceptions data is useful for identifying problems that may not be life threatening but cause substantial decreases in quality of life. The perceptions of health needs of at least three groups can contribute to an understanding of women's health needs.

Community perceptions. The perceptions of health needs expressed by women themselves can provide unique information. In New Zealand, Walton and colleagues (1988) asked 2000 randomly selected women to comment on their health services. Forty five per cent of the women indicated the need for changes in the health services. The most common requests were for changes to hospital services where delays, centralisation and referral patterns were perceived as problems, and in general practice, particularly doctor-patient communication and the cost of some aspects of health care.

Redman et al. (1988) undertook a survey of a randomly selected community sample of women. They provided the 125 women interviewed with a list of health problems and asked them to indicate the three problems with which they would most have liked help with in the past six months. The proportion of women indicating each problem listed among their top three is shown in the left hand column of Table 3.4. The most commonly listed problems were weight, stress and money problems. Smoking, caring for sick and elderly relatives, menstrual problems and the cost of medical care were also frequently mentioned as priority problems.

This method of assessing needs has some disadvantages. It is more likely to detect common low level problems. While many may have had the opportunity to feel stressed or to have menstrual problems over a weekly period very few women will have experienced problems such as breast or cervical cancer.

Lobby groups. Priority areas may also be established by consensus among special interest groups. The process used by the NSW Women's Health Policy Review Committee (1985) is an example of this process. The committee placed newspaper advertisements which requested submissions from community and consumer groups, organisations and individuals on health care services. The advertisements mentioned work pressures, family planning advice, smoking and drug use and friendlier more effective health care services as questions which would be considered. The Committee received 244 submissions and held 27 community consultations. This method of assessing priorities appears to be valid because those groups who are dissatisfied with existing care have the opportunity to argue their case.

The review nominated 279 priorities for women's health. Because of its consensus process, the review committee could not provide a quantitative assessment to select major priorities from its lengthy list. It did however propose that particular attention be paid to issues relating to gynaecological health, menopause, psychotropic use, alcohol and smoking.

Lobby groups can however provide a biased view of the true needs in the community. It seems likely that the views of the more articulate and better organised group will be over-represented. It might be argued that the lobby group method of setting priorities transfers power from the medical hierarchy to a group of relatively privileged women.

Health care providers. Reviewing the opinions of health care providers is the traditional method of establishing health care priorities. However, it has been argued that health care providers are a particularly inappropriate group for deciding on priorities in women's health for several reasons. First, it is unlikely that the views of health care providers will adequately reflect areas in which women are dissatisfied with care. For example, although obstetricians and gynaecologists are

Table 3.4: percentage of women including each health problem as a personal priority

Life threatening health	Personal	Chronic health problem	Personal
1. Heart disease	6.3	35. Arthritis	8.6
2. Lung disease	6.3	36. Diabetes	3.1
3. Cervical cancer	0.8		
4. Breast Cancer	1.6	**Menstrual problems**	
5. Other cancer	3.9	37. Problems with periods	10.2
6. Road traffic accident	3.9	38. Premenstrual tension	7.0
7. Other accidents	1.6	39. Menopause problems	2.3
8. Suicide or suicide attempts	0		
		Reproductive problems	
Gynaecological problems		40. Problems in becoming pregnant	3.1
9. Thrush	1.6	41. Pregnancy complications	1.6
10. STDs	0.8	42. Miscarriage	0.8
11. UTIs	1.6	43. Abortion	0
12. Problems with womb or uterus	1.6	44. Childbirth problems	1.6
		45. Contraceptive problems	
Parenting problems			
13. Problems with a new baby	3.1	**Relationship problems**	
14. Problems with child's health	3.1	46. With partner or husband	6.3
15. Baby or child feeding problems	0.8	47. With other family members	3.9
16. Child behaviour problems	4.7	48. Lack of interest in sex	3.1
17. Parenting problems	0	49. Caring for elderly relative	10.2
18 Childcare/babysitting problems	3.9		
		Health risks	
Psychological problems		50. Smoking	11.7
19. Anxiety	7.0	51. Drinking	0
20. Depression	9.4	52. Overweight	16.4
21. Stress	16.4	53. Lack of exercise	5.5
22. Tiredness	7.0	54. Using tranquilisers	1.6
23. Not feeling confident	3.9		
24. Disturbed sleep	8.6	**Work problems**	
25. Loneliness	3.1	55. Unemployment	5.5
26. Feeling isolated	2.3	56. Job satisfaction	3.9
27. Not enough self-time	9.4	57. Combining work with parenting	3.1
Living Problems		**Medical care**	
28. Money Problems	14.8	58. Dissatisfaction with quality	8.6
29. Housing problems	0	59. Poor access	4.7
30. Transport problems	3.1	60. Cost	10.2
Violence			
31. Rape	1.6		
32. Incest	1.6		
33. Sexual harrassment	0.8		
34. Physical violence	1.6		

If You Don't Like It ...

'Dale Street' is a small regional women's health centre in the western suburbs of Adelaide. In 1987, the centre became involved with local residents who were concerned about pollution in their neighbourhood and its effects on their health. On the surface, this activity appeared a departure from the traditional concerns of the women's health movement. But the philosophical framework of the movement, and its tradition of speaking out for change, enabled and encouraged such a development to occur.

The first women's health centre in South Australia was established at Hindmarsh in 1975 under the federal Community Health Program. Dale Street, located in Port Adelaide, is one of four government-funded women's health centres operating in South Australia. All are managed and staffed by women.

Other centres were founded in the mid-1970s in Sydney, Darwin and Perth. In Melbourne, a women's health resource centre was established without government funding. All operate as collectives and are seen as radical and anti-establishment especially by the medical establishment.

As in other states, women's health centres in South Australia emerged from the women's movement of the 1960s and 1970s. Women came together to share their experiences, and learnt that these often were at variance with popular and public views of their lives. They also recognised that they had important statements to make about the changes they wanted in the world around them, and a right to be heard.

Key issues for women centred on their right to have control over their own bodies, to make their own decisions about pregnancy and childbirth, to be given the information they needed to make choices about their health care and to challenge widely held medical opinions about so-called female pathology. Building on their experiences, they understood the unequal power relations in society and the significance of the social as well as the individual environment.

There have been significant changes and development since these early days and difficult struggles. In South Australia, centres have lost some of their radical feminist edge, and have moved closer to the bureaucracy. They have gained greater acceptance and respectability and have become involved in policy making while continuing to provide a range of gynaecologically based medical care and other services, including information, education and community development. The involvement of the Adelaide Women's Community Health Centre and the Working Women's Centre in campaigning for and with women suffering repetition strain injuries has been an important development in the 1980s, bringing to the forefront the health issues of women in the paid workforce. During this time broad alliances have also been formed with other community organisation and unions.

It is this background and these principles — of access to information, the right to participate in making decisions which affect our lives and the belief that the health and well being of people is shaped by the environment in which we live — which have been so important in shaping the development of women's health. The impact of such principles has been strengthened by a willingness to be outward looking, building links with other relevant organisation.

Dale Street has been built on this experience and has consciously fostered strong community links. Local women have ensured an emphasis on the provision of health information and an acknowledgement of the validity of each woman's experience in being treated by staff at the centre. On the management committee local women have accepted and strengthened the commitment to primary prevention. In planning new programs, both workers and management committee members have raised for consideration the health issues and concerns that appear important locally. Its goals reflect its understanding of health and well being as critically affected by social circumstances and relations.

The experience of local women and the community led to Dale Street's involvement in environmental health activities. Over a period of time, centre workers became concerned at the high rate of respiratory problems that were reported by women. At about the same time contact was made with a group of people who, for some years, had battled with nearby industries about problems such as factory emissions, dust, vehicle noise and emergency procedures in the event of an accident. These residents lived literally across the road from a ribbon of large industries. They grew angry about the lack of effective action and fearful of the possible effects on their health.

Other people in nearby areas were also worried by the proximity of industry to housing. In 1985, a environmental group was formed as a result of concerns about a spill of copper chromium arsenate in the Port River. A major spill of chlorine gas some months later heightened awareness about the dangers of this potentially disastrous accident. Had the wind been blowing towards the houses instead of towards the river, an evacuation of residents would have been necessary, and people's lives could have been at risk.

As a way of assessing the extent of resident concern about their health problems, the centre employed a local woman on a short-term basis to run a survey. The results of this were published in a report entitled *If You Don't Like It, Move,* which describes the anxieties and fears of a community that believes that the environment is affecting its health. The findings and recommendations of the report were presented at a public meeting which was attended by over 200 people, including representatives from industry and state and local government.

As a consequence, the South Australian Health Commission included the region as one of a small number of pilot projects in local environmental health management planning. This process involves the identification and assessment of known environmental pollutants and their health effects, and the development of an action plan to address those problems. It has been an exciting development, bringing together government experts, local government health inspectors and surveyors, community health workers and residents. The action plan is not yet completed, and progress towards it is often slow and difficult. In spite of the frustrations it has great potential.

While it was the direct link with local women that provided the immediate stimulus to Dale Street to take action, it has been the philosophical framework within which the centre operates which has led it to identify environmental health as an issue which it should address. As a women's health centre, it could have decided to take no direct action because it did not only affect women. It was, however, an issue which was raised by women and which affected women's health and well being. As the social and cultural environment have long been regarded as vitally important to women's health, it was a simple extension to acknowledge also the physical environment.

It is sometimes argued that women's health has moved from the radical sixties into the mainstream eighties. A part of this argument involves a recognition that women's health has had considerable influence because its methods work. In areas such as client information and community participation, its techniques have been generalised to a wider range of organisations. The movement is certainly closer to the bureaucracy now, and its skills in, for instance, policy development and planning are used by the bureaucracy. The balance between maintaining momentum as agents of change while still having influence and recognition at a bureaucratic level can be a delicate one.

A look at the priority issues identified in the National Women's Health Policy shows, however, that many of the reasons which led women to set up women's health centres still remain crucial. While environmental health became a focus at Dale Street, the essential services of the centre (such as information provision, gynaecologically based health care and an approach to problems such as domestic violence that includes a social and preventive context), are still much in demand. The struggle for accessible abortion services is still being waged, and access to information remains a vital issue to women.

Women's health has always been about change. This example of environmental health action demonstrates how the early principles of the women's health movement continue to provide a basis for new arenas of action.

Jocelyn Auer and Clare Shuttleworth, *Australian Society,* February 1990.

consulted about their priorities for women's reproductive health, these same doctors may be the target of women's dissatisfaction with existing care. Second, the priorities nominated by health care providers may be biased towards their area of expertise, that is, they may be more likely to select health problems which they know about or see on a regular basis. They may also select those problems which promote or maintain their discipline. Finally, they cannot know about the burden of illness from a particular problem at the community level — they know only about those problems with which women believe the doctor may be able to help.

PRIORITIES

It is evident that there is an urgent need to develop more sophisticated methods of accessing community and other views of health priorities. There is a need to ensure that even consensus processes yield clear priorities for action. The collection of more information about what women themselves consider to be priorities is of obvious importance.

REFERENCES

Australian Bureau of Statistics (1978). *Australian health survey 1977-1978*, Cat. no. 4311.0, ABS, Canberra.

Australian Bureau of Statistics (1983). *Australian health survey*, Cat. no. 4311.0, ABS, Canberra.

Australian Bureau of Statistics (1984). *Social indicators Australia No. 4*, Cat. no. 4101.0, ABS, Canberra.

Australian Bureau of Statistics (1986). *Hospital in-patients NSW*, Cat. no. 43061, ABS, Sydney.

Australian Bureau of Statistics (1988). *Australian demographic statistics*, Cat. no. 3101.0, ABS, Canberra.

Australian Bureau of Statistics (1988). *Causes of death Australia*, Cat. no. 3308.0, ABS, Canberra.

Dickinson, J.A., Wiggers, J., Leeder, S.R. & Sanson-Fisher, R.W. (1989). General practitioners' detection of patients' smoking status, *The medical journal of Australia*, 150, 420–426.

Mitchell, H. & Medley, G. (1987). Age trends in Pap smear usage, 1971–1986, *Community health studies*, 11, 183–185.

National Heart Foundation (1983). *A profile of Australians, a summary of the National Heart Foundation risk factor prevalence study*, Report No. 2.

Redman, S., Hennrikus, D.J., Bowman, J.A. & Sanson-Fisher, R.W. (1988). Assessing women's health needs, *The medical journal of Australia*, 148, 123–127.

Tabar, L., Fagerberg, G., Duffy, S.W. & Day, N.E. (1989). The Swedish 2 country trial of mammographic screening for breast cancer: recent results and calculation of benefit. *Journal of epidemiology & community health*, 43, 107–114.

Waldron, I. (1983). Sex differences in illness incidence, prognosis and mortality: issues and evidence, *Social science & medicine*, 17 (6), 1107–1123.

Walton, V.A., Roman-Clarkson, S.E. & Mullen, P.E. (1988). Improvements urban and rural women wish to see in their health care services, *New Zealand medical journal*, 101, 80–82.

Wingard, D. (1984). Sex differentials in mortality, morbidity and lifestyle, *Annual review of public health*, 5, 433–458.

Women's Health Policy Review Committee (1985). *Women's health services in NSW*, Sydney, NSW Government Printer.

4 Women and Health Promotion

Rapid technological developments in the twentieth century have changed the face of health care for women. This is particularly true in the practice of medicine e.g. obstetrics. Early recognition of patterns of illness has led to an increased visibility of diseases. In chapter one, we discussed how diseases were removed from the realm of women's influence. Superstition and uncertainty diminished as diseases were made more quantifiable. Foucault (1973) argues that through this development, disease became the validator of medicine. This process has now extended to encompass the causation of disease. Any residual uncertainty left over from the era of witches and midwives is now clarified by an approach which is called multifactorial and has measurable biological, psychological and social components.

DIAGNOSIS AND TREATMENT

Medical attention has focused on the more easily measurable techniques and methods of diagnosis. Laboratory methods, X rays, imaging techniques and, more recently, computerised systems are the fundamentals of this assessment. Whilst these improvements in diagnostic technology have allowed the earlier and in some cases, more accurate, diagnosis of many conditions, cost has often prohibited their widespread use amongst women.

Increasing sophistication and visibility of diagnosis has led to a demand for accompanying effective treatments. Although methods of treatment have been developed, the capacity to alter the course of advanced disease states has been limited. Cure is no longer the end point of a treatment intervention, e.g. as antibiotics have been in the cure of bacterial infections.

The promise of the new diagnostic technology was sold to women in three ways which directly related to the provision of health care services and indirectly, if at all, to their needs as consumers:

1) diseases would become more easily explained and therefore, more easily accessible to scientific analysis and solution;
2) the enormous development and operational costs of this technology would be recouped by the financial advantages of early and more accurate diagnosis, and
3) the basis of medical practice, i.e. the relationship between diagnosis and treatment, would be strengthened.

To have any medical significance, diagnostic sophistication would have to lead to treatment sophistication. This, in turn, would result in diminished morbidity and mortality. Women would benefit by being freed from illness. Communities would benefit by not having to carry the financial, social and political burdens of women's illness.

PREVENTION

The promise of freedom from illness has not been fulfilled. A chasm has developed between diagnosis and cure. Cure is no longer the expected end product of many diagnosis/treatment pathways. Other outcomes are being recognised, including chronic illness, incurable disease and disability. Thus mortality may have been diminished but morbidity for women has increased (see chapter three).

Where the sophistication of diagnostic technology has been accessible to women, there has not always been an accompanying level of refined treatment and management. For example, osteoarthritis, an ever-increasing problem for women, can now be identified in its early stages through radiodensitrometry. However, the progression of this condition can be at best slowed, at worst unchanged.

The end of the medical pathway could no longer be called a certain cure. This growing mismatch between diagnosis and treatment has led women to look for new strategies. Attention has focused on the beginning of the pathway. The concept of prevention of disease has achieved greater prominence. The belief is that disease and illness can be prevented. This is an even more comfortable notion than cure. Once again, the promise has been that community and women's morbidity would be lessened.

The link with illness has meant that prevention has remained a domain of medical practice. Brown (1985) has described three levels which relate directly to the medical field:

• primary prevention refers to measures taken before illness begins, e.g. rubella immunisation;

- secondary prevention is concerned with limiting disease by early disease detection, e.g. screening for cervical cancer;
- tertiary prevention refers to attempts to stop deterioration, e.g. rehabilitation programs for women with osteoarthritis.

These strategies have been directed particularly to health care providers. But all three levels of prevention involve a more active role in health care for women than has previously existed. The identification of health risks, and the utilisation of intervention measures to reduce the risk of illness, requires the co-operative efforts of both women as consumers and both men and women as providers. Webster (1978) argues that the response of the medical community has been at best slow, at worst token, despite significant opportunities at all levels.

Within the context of primary care, both groups have been working at readjusting the balance of responsibility for prevention. The *National women's health policy* (1989) recommends that a comprehensive and accessible network of primary health care services should be available for all women, as well as access to high quality secondary and tertiary services when required. Women are being offered and are taking more responsibility for the prevention of their illness. Communication and health education techniques have been the major instruments in this task. This new found dynamic has not been easy for medical practitioners, who have been trained in the diagnosis/treatment/cure pathway. The *National women's health policy* acknowledges the need for professional training for all practitioners in the area of women's health. All curricula should address:

- the health status of women;
- the health care needs of women;
- specific clinical skills relating to the health of women;
- high level interpersonal skills;
- issues of dignity and privacy; and
- the elimination of discriminatory practices.

Pap smears — how reliable are they?

Pauline Whittaker is a bubbly 42-year-old mother of three sons. In January this year she had a radical hysterectomy which removed her uterus, cervix, and some of her lymph nodes, because she had been diagnosed as having invasive cancer of the cervix. The diagnosis came as a surprise because Pauline, a trained nurse, had been having regular Pap smears for most of her adult life. As a nurse, she knew that Pap smears were a woman's best protection against cervical cancer because they can detect treatable and curable pre-cancerous changes in the cervix before they become malignant. In the 12 months before her hysterectomy Pauline had a smear which indicated inflammation but showed no abnormality when the test was repeated a short time later. A subsequent smear indicated inflammation, although Pauline had no symptoms of infection. Investigation by a gynaecologist finally revealed invasive cancer.

Unlike Pauline, Penny Stoyles and Christine Evely were not lucky enough to have had children when invasive cancer of the cervix was diagnosed. In their late twenties, both women had hysterectomies as the only possible life-saving treatment. The histories of their disease are not identical but they share the worrying fact that regular Pap smears did not detect cancerous changes in the cervix until it was too late for conservative treatment to prevent the development of cancer. Drastic surgical removal of most of their reproductive organs was the only possible course of action. Penny and Christine are both members of the Cervical Cancer Support Group in Victoria, which assists women in coming to terms with the effects of their disease.

The Pap test is unique in cancer detection because its use can detect pre-cancerous changes in the cervix before they become malignant and life threatening. These pre-cancerous changes can be easily treated by a number of fairly simple techniques, including removal by laser, freezing, heat application and conventional surgery. Pre-cancer can be cured, preventing the subsequent development of cancer of the cervix, drastic treatment, and even loss of life.

All you need to do, so the argument goes, is have your regular smears done, and you will not be one of the 1000 new cases of cervical cancer detected annually in Australia, and the 350 deaths which occur as a result.

But the experiences of Pauline, Penny and Christine suggest that perhaps it is not quite so simple. Perhaps women need to know more about the subject, to ensure they are getting maximum benefit from their smears.

There has been intense debate in Australia recently about the effectiveness of Pap smears as a screening tool.

It is sometimes asserted that health-conscious young women may be over-screened — that is, they have more Pap smears than they really need. Many other women, including those in the high-risk older age groups, have too few.

Not only is there confusion in the general community about how frequently Pap smears should be performed, but disagreement within the medical profession is vociferous.

The argument is complicated by considerations of the cost effectiveness of possible screening programs. It's all very well to spend millions of dollars screening women for cancer of the cervix, but will it actually save lives?

Dr Heather Mitchell, an epidemiologist with the Victorian Cytology (Gynaecology) Service, says new cases of cervical cancer could be reduced to 150 a year, and deaths to 50, 'if we were doing things properly'.

'Doing things properly' is the hard part. Underpinning many of the arguments about screening, and in particular the view that triennial Pap smears would be both cost-effective and efficacious, is the assumption that the smear test itself is reliable.

The truth is that Pap smears, which undeniably have saved lives, are in fact subject to considerable error. The error rate of the smears themselves is not nearly as publicly debated as other aspects of the screening issue, such as why women fail to request smears — perhaps because it is the health professionals themselves who are responsible for it.

Anxiety about medico-legal issues sometimes surfaces when the error rate is discussed because it is possible that women may attempt to hold the doctor or pathologist legally responsible if they fail to perform their task properly.

Pap smears are either negative (no abnormality), or positive (indicating an abnormality of some kind, but not necessarily pre-cancer).

False positives will cause anxiety of course, but false negatives are the real concern. Apart from things like clerical mixups, there are two main areas in which error, or at least lack of expertise, knowledge and professionalism, can influence the smear to give an incorrect result.

The first, and most likely, area where an error can occur is in the taking of the smear itself. Dr Julienne Grace, of Sydney's Royal Prince Alfred Hospital, chairs the Cytology Quality Assurance Program run by the Royal College of Pathologists of Australasia. She estimates that as much as two-thirds of error is attributable to poor sampling. There can be too few cells, the smears can be contaminated by blood or infection, or the sample may not have been 'fixed' properly, meaning that the cells have not been effectively preserved.

Taking Pap smears is not necessarily easy ... The statistics which Dr Grace collects through the Royal Prince Alfred Hospital's pathology unit show a wide disparity from clinic to clinic, and person to person, in the quality of the smears collected. Importantly, there is a great capacity for improvement with education and training.

One rural clinic which had an alarming 23 per cent adequacy rate one month, had lifted its game to 55 per cent three months later. A clinic for post-menopausal women, who are anatomically much more difficult to sample than younger women, achieved a consistently high rate of between 85 and 92 per cent, which Dr Grace said was attributable to the dedication and skill of the doctor who took the smears.

Dr Colin Laverty, a pathologist whose practice specialises in gynaecological cytology, confirms this view, saying that the percentage of smears which contains endocervical cells varies enormously from doctor to doctor. A few specialist gynaecologists were poor at taking smears, despite wide experience. Others had excellent success rates, as did many general practitioners, who may have had a lot less practice.

How many women are actually ever told that their smears are inadequate (and that the time, inconvenience and cost of a repeat smear is necessary) is anyone's guess, but you can bet it isn't all of them.

A woman cannot be sure herself unless she's shown the pathology report, a far from common practice, although women have the right to know what is contained in it.

Inadequate smears can be made by anyone, because the technique is a manual one conducted by human beings. There will always be a proportion of women, like some who already had treatment to the cervix, in whom it is very difficult to obtain endocervical cells.

But this is not for the majority, and the point is whether the clinician keeps this knowledge from the woman, fearing either a question of legal responsibility, a reputation for incompetence, or, and this is worse, because he or she does not understand the implications of the pathology report itself. This last is a distinct possibility since it is not obligatory for doctors, or other health practitioners, to keep up with the latest in scientific knowledge contained in the medical journals.

Much has improved in the world of Pap smears in recent years. The College of Pathologists is conducting an ongoing quality assurance program with its members, and currently recommends that the best smear is achieved through the use of both a spatula and a brush, rather than just one instrument.

Both the Royal Australian College of General Practitioners and the Royal Australian College of Obstetricians and Gynaecologists distribute information and education to their members about changes in knowledge in the area. Dr David Knight, representing the general practitioners, adds that if a woman's doctor refuses to show her the pathology result 'she should get an opinion from another doctor'.

In conjunction with State health departments, the Federal Department of Community Services and Health is conducting pilot programs throughout Australia to 'investigate the feasibility and cost-effectiveness of providing a co-ordinated and comprehensive nationwide program for cervical cancer screening'.

Until the reliability of Pap smears can be demonstrated, the debate about whether they should be performed annually, or on a far more cost effective triennial basis, is likely to remain an emotional one. The chances of compensating for a possible error in sampling or testing increase with the frequency of the smears.

Dr Julienne Grace says: 'So long as 50 per cent of the smears may not be sampling the appropriate area, then in the current light of knowledge in this country we must continue to do annual smears, just to keep cervical cancer at the rate we have now.

'I believe that if we don't do what we are doing now, the incidence will start to rise, but we won't see it for five years and then we'll realise we've made a mistake. That could be as many as 3000 women in Australia, over five years, who will have died unnecessarily.'

The unreliability of some smears does not justify any woman deciding not to have them. On the contrary, Pap smears are the best tool available to prevent the development of cervical cancer and the unnecessary deaths which can result. Smear takers, and the laboratories that test the smears, must be pressured to reduce the rate of error, so much of which is avoidable, and allow Pap smears to achieve the best possible level of performance.

Margo Beasley, *The Australian Women's Weekly*, November 1989

SHARING HEALTH CARE

The *National women's health policy* (1989) recognises that reorientation of the conventional health care system is insufficient. Special women's health services are needed to examine new issues and develop new models of services which can then influence existing general health services.

Through this process there has been a gradual shift in responsibilities between providers and the women who use these services. This may be natural evolution and/or the result of medical inertia. Women have become more active in the co-operative management of their illness. Their expectations have changed. Irwin and Brown (1981) argue that the move from preoccupation with the treatment of illness to the prevention of illness requires not only a reconsideration of the present health care networks, but also the promotion of health within these contexts. No longer is an expectation of the health practitioner curing illness or delivering an end point sufficient. Practitioners are expected to intervene at a starting point.

HEALTH PROMOTION

The body of knowledge and the range of activities that constitute health promotion are still under exploration and consolidation. Recently, attempts have been made to mould the concepts of health promotion into a framework which is already accepted within the health care sector.

In the same way that she identified three levels of prevention which were disease orientated and related to the medical field, Brown (1985) has identified three levels of health promotion which are unrelated to the medical field, but related to the health field:

- primary health promotion to eradicate health-related risks;
- secondary health promotion to raise the quality of life; and
- tertiary health promotion to bring about enduring social change.

The process of implementing this content within the context of the individual, the community and society has received an international commitment. A charter for action was produced at the WHO First International Conference on Health Promotion in Ottawa in 1986. Known as the *Ottawa Charter*, it defines both the process and content of health promotion.

Health is defined in the broadest of terms. It is not the objective of living, but rather the resource for everyday life. Implicit in this definition is the notion that the health status of women goes beyond illness and that it is possible to enable women to affect changes in their current health status.

It is clear that the *Charter*, by remaining broad, does not intend to pre-empt future possible directions of health promotion. Its aim is to promote and validate health promotion action. In fact, so broad are the definitions that a new taxonomy has developed under the umbrella of the notion of health promotion. Health protection, health advancement, health education and health maintenance are just a few of the new descriptors.

The Charter defines five broad categories of action:

1) an individual approach, involving the development of personal skills. Through the provision of information, health education and programs to enhance life skills, women would be able to exercise more control over their own health and make choices conducive to health.

Implicit in this approach is the role of education and personal development in health. The empowering of women with health knowledge and the means to affect health changes, it is deemed, would lead them to greater control over their own health. This progression cannot occur in isolation and must proceed in concert with broader objectives.

2) a community approach, involving the development of local strategies to support the processes and empowering strategies which assist individual women.

At this level health promotion becomes an agent of social change affecting more than just the environment of individual women. Discrete notions coalesce into community concepts to shape further change. The pathway is bidirectional. The community strategy of health education can be used to develop and support the health actions and behaviours of individual women.

3) an ecological approach, acknowledging the complex interrelationships between health of women and the environments in which they live and work.

This perspective of health acknowledges the strong links between domestic and work environments. It incorporates the intersectoral relationships between industry and the communities from which the workforce is drawn and to which the outputs of industry are provided.

4) a health sector approach, which acknowledges the integral role health services can play at all levels of health care. With this approach, the brief of the health sector would be expanded to embrace the growing notions of health promotion. The reorientation of health services advocated in this Charter has major implications for women in Australia. The Charter implicitly validates the role of the general practitioner taking on a community and health promoting agenda as well as an individual case approach and the treatment of sickness.

5) an organisational approach which takes health beyond health care. This would involve initiatives in legislation, fiscal policy, taxation and social structures.

The overall goal of health promotion is to foster greater equity at local, national and international levels.

HEALTH FOR ALL

The Australian response to the Ottawa Charter was a Health Targets and Implementation (Health For All) Committee under the auspices of the Australian Health Ministers' Advisory Council. This committee was to present the findings of its report at the Adelaide conference. Initially, the committee was to determine the areas in which health goals and targets were to be set. A large and unavoidably uneven compendium of goals and targets, Health for All Australians (1988) were defined under the following areas:

- population groups;
- major causes of illness; and
- death and risk factors.

Later in the same year a smaller, more addressable group of five health targets were identified as priorities for action. Whilst one of these targets was directly related to the health of a specific population, the target group was older people not women. The promotion of health for women was indirectly addressed under the target of prevention of specific cancers.

The complementary task of identifying the implementation targets for health promotion was left to the National Project Implementation Teams. However, the committee did identify the structural changes necessary. They included planning and policy development, health workforce education and training and consumer/community participation. Agreements to provide financial incentives to promote health and, most importantly, to support health promotion in primary health care were reached between the commonwealth government and the state governments. This indicates a recognition of the importance of primary health care in the promotion of health. However, the exact role and function of the primary health care sector in relation to the health of women was not defined.

The argument for not including women as a target group centred on the fact that there was a separate initiative in the area of women's health. This project was the development of a *National women's health policy*. Thus the health of women was marginalised and has since remained separate from mainstream activities of health promotion. If through the process of validating health promotion women become alienated from mainstream decisions about their own health and also from the broader arena of society's decision making processes, there will be an increasing tendency to see them as dependent. Their illness will become more prominent and attention will once again focus on the treatment and prevention of these illness.

Despite the WHO validation of the adoption of health promotion strategies for women, little definitive research has been carried out into practical methods for integrating these strategies. Kelly's (1988) program of addressing seven lifestyle change factors (amount of food, type of food, stress, exercise, smoking, alcohol and seat belt use) shows some promise but it is not particularly related to women. Frame (1986) remains sceptical and questions the efficacy of many available methods.

For women it is not easy to share ideas about health with their providers when the relationship is so overwhelmed with chronic and acute illness — its prevention and treatment. Freeman (1987) goes one step further by suggesting that health practitioners avoid affecting change. She outlines the difficulty of introducing health promotion exchanges into the medical consultation. She goes further to suggest that health promotion is a 'troublesome' topic for both providers and their women patients and that both employ conversational strategies to distance these topics from the rest of the interview. In a pessimistic way she supports the notion that health and illness content in a consultation must be separated.

Freeman's strategy to overcome the problem of introducing the health promotion agenda preempts the notion of separate health promotion consultations. In this way, she argues, the difficulties encountered in introducing the topic would be minimised.

THE FUTURE

The supposed new emphasis on promoting the health of women is not new at all. It really reflects a return to the early days of health care where the approach was more integrated and women centred. The process of defining health for women has proved difficult under the constraining parameters of illness and cure. Sontag (1977) highlights the conflicts between health and illness for women

> Illness is the night-side of life, a more onerous citizenship. Everyone who is born holds dual citizenship, in the kingdom (sic) of the well and in the kingdom of the sick. Although we all prefer to use only the good passport, sooner or later each of us is obliged, at least for a spell, to identify ourselves of citizens of that other place.

Even more difficult has been the establishment of sustainable programs. In Australia the *National women's health policy* provides a template for structural change — very little of which has been implemented. Women's health in Australia is trapped by the three Rs:

'riting — much has been written;
reading — not much has been read; and
'rithmetic — all of it is too expensive.

For the circle to be complete, lip service should be abandoned. The legitimate health concerns of women need to be incorporated at all levels of the health care system. Women and health committees need to be established within state and federal departments of health where they are directly responsible to the minister in charge. The primary task of these committees is to ensure that all projects undertaken by the departments have a women's brief. In the private sector, strategies should follow those that have been developed for occupational health and equal opportunity. Health industries vying for government favour or contract should be requested to provide functional briefs on their strategies concerning women's health.

Evaluation and monitoring should be integral to these initiatives to ensure that processes are not duplicated and sustainable change is achieved. In the areas of education, welfare, transport and social policy, women's health should be integrated through similar strategies.

CASE STUDY

The Minister for Health, Dr Blewett, was addressing participants to the Healthy Public Policy Conference sponsored by the Australian Department of Health and the World Health Organisation in 1987. Australia's blueprint for Health for All by the Year 2000 — the espoused goal of WHO — was being presented to the packed lecture theatre of national and international delegates.

The press were present — and so were a delegation of Aboriginal women. Unannounced and uninvited they quietly took the podium as the Minister spoke of special initiatives in Aboriginal health, and passionately but proudly demanded funding for the Aboriginal controlled program of obstetric care — The Congress Alukura by the Grandmother's Law.

The papers they distributed described the beginning of the Central Aboriginal Congress in June 1973, and how

> in 1979 Aboriginal people began undertaking their own research and study. Health business was to achieve a redefinition of health and to clarify the process required to improve Aboriginal health in the Centre...It was during this time that Aboriginal women began to describe their reasons for delaying antenatal check-ups and their lonely frightening and shaming experiences during hospitalised childbirth, and the disruption that it brought to traditional midwifery and related ceremonial practices. They advocated the establishment of a 'birthing centre' that would assure ease and comfort through a continuation of traditional practices.
>
> Aboriginal women say that Aboriginal control is the key issue in the reduction of Aboriginal mortality and morbidity and that by developing services in a more culturally appropriate way, including the most elementary aspect of culture, which is language, Aboriginal women would be able to ensure the survival of their babies.
>
> We are offering a practical solution to how the maintenance of Aboriginal Law can provide a stable and cultural base from which women can fuse aspects of traditional ways of life with the realities of modern life.
>
> The Congress Alukura has a commitment to shifting the emphasis of the health system significantly towards the promotion of health and wellbeing through a social view of health. This involves a view to which patterns of health and illness are clearly linked to social, cultural, political and economic factors.

Their stand highlighted the need for women's health issues to be given priority in discussions about health promotion, and healthy public policy, and their voice was strengthened by a formal endorsement of their proposal by the conference.

It is an important step, but a standing ovation at an international conference is not enough unless some change follows...

REFERENCES

Brown, V.A. (1985). Towards an epidemiology of health: a basis for planning community health programs, *Health policy*, 4, 331–340.

Foucault, M. (1973). *The birth of the clinic*, Tavistock Publications, London.

Frame, P.S. (1986). A critical review of adult health maintenance, Parts 1,2,3 & 4, *Journal of family practice*; 22, 341–346, 417–426, 511–520; 23, 29–42.

Freeman, S.H. (1987). Health promotion talk in family practice encounters, *Journal of social science in medicine*, 25 (8), 961–966.

Health For All Australians Committee to Australian Health Ministers (1988). *Report by health target and implementation (Health for All) committee*, Commonwealth Department of Health, Canberra.

Irwin, R.P. & Brown, V.A. (1981). Personal care and public good, *Australian family physician*, 10, 536–541.

Kelly, R.B. (1988). Controlled trial of time efficient method of health promotion, *American journal of preventive medicine*, 4, 200–207.

National Women's Health Policy (1989). *National women's health policy: advancing women's health in Australia*, AGPS, Canberra.

Ottawa Charter for Health Promotion (1987). *Bulletin of the Pan American Health Organisation*, 21, 200–204.

Sontag, S. (1977). *Illness as metaphor*, Penguin, New York.

Webster, I.W. (1978). *Preventive medicine*, School of Community Medicine, University of New South Wales.

5 Women as Providers and Consumers of Health Care

This chapter discusses the role of women in the health care system in an Australian context and explores issues relevant to women both as providers and consumers of health care. Often aspects of the roles of women in health care are ignored, particularly women as providers in the home environment. In addition, issues are raised concerning the low status of women health care providers and women's lack of power within this system. Reasons for these imbalances are explored.

THE HEALTH CARE WORKFORCE

Women are the major providers of health care in Australia. This statement is an accurate description of the two levels in which women provide health care: paid and unpaid.

The health industry is the second largest employer of women in Australia today, after the retail industry. Whilst women do not form the majority of decision makers in health care, they certainly constitute the majority of workers. According to Census data (1986), women comprise 76 per cent of health industry employees. Seventy-five per cent of these women are professionals, distributed in the following proportions:

- 93 per cent of occupational therapists;
- 92.5 per cent of nurses;
- 84 per cent of physiotherapists;
- 71 per cent of social workers;
- 25 per cent of medical practitioners;
- 22 per cent of optometrists;
- 15 per cent of chiropractors and osteopaths; and
- 13.5 per cent of dentists.

The growth areas for women health care professionals are:

- medical practitioners;
- dentists;
- optometrists;
- radiographers;
- physiotherapists; and
- occupational therapists.

However, while there is an increase in the number of women medical practitioners — the Commonwealth Department of Community Services and Health's Medical Manpower Survey of 1984 estimated that by the year 1990 42 per cent of all medical graduates will be women — women are not well represented in the medical specialties. For example, there are only 414 female consultant physicians compared with 2393 males (15 per cent), and 105 female obstetricians and gynaecologists compared with 1068 males (9 per cent) according to the Australian Medical Association.

An effect of the concentration of women in some professions was labelled 'feminisation of the workforce' by the manpower survey of 1984. This process has profound effects on the workforce; usually lower wages and salaries. In 1981, one in three female doctors earned less than $8000 a year, compared with one in ten male doctors (Saltman 1989). The 1986 census data revealed that nearly one third of general practitioners were earning less than $30 000. It is probably no coincidence that nearly one third of general practitioners are women. It seems that women doctors would be better off employed in the care of their own children.

In the area of health management, women are underemployed. Census data (1986) reveal that only 2 per cent of general managers, e.g. medical superintendents, chief executives and hospital administrators, are women, but it should be noted that this figure rather tellingly excludes Directors of Nursing.

The data on professionals and health managers do not include the vast numbers of workers in semi-skilled and unskilled jobs, e.g. kitchen hands, ward clerks and cleaners, the majority of whom are women. In the lower paid, lower status areas, women from non English speaking backgrounds are more likely to predominate because they are less likely to have qualifications to obtain more skilled work (ABS 1986). However, there are a variety of jobs specifically suited for non English speaking background women and Aboriginal and Torres Strait Islander women, including interpreting services, information officers and hospital liaison officers.

Regrettably, the diversity of roles has tended to polarise women in the health care workforce. The tendency to lateral violence of women against women is a growing concern. When women assume male centred frameworks and operate within them, there is a danger from what Alford (1972) calls 'dynamics without change'. As women workers in health care ascend the ladders to power they become fewer in number. They are more exposed to the entrenched hierarchies. They often decide that adopting the current status quo is the pathway of least resistance. Women in senior positions become part of the old boy's club. There, these 'successful' few appear to be socialised to believe that their attainment of these positions has been only as a direct result of their skill and effort which is equal to that of their male counterparts but much greater than those of other women. This leads to the erroneous assumption that only a few women are good, bright and clever enough to hold down these positions and that, by inference, all other women workers in health care must be less than adequate.

Furler (1985) argues that the lack of women in positions of power and influence in the health care system has far greater structural implications. She argues that this imbalance has contributed to the situation where mainstream health services are not necessarily appropriate to women's needs.

Women in medicine

A father and son have a car accident. The father is killed, the son badly injured. He is rushed to hospital by ambulance for emergency surgery. The surgeon, donning mask and gloves, runs in to the operating theatre ready to act, but, after taking one look at the boy, says 'I can't operate. That's my son.'

The most extreme example of the masculinisation of the few women who ascend the powerful professional ladder is that the term health professional is often equated with doctor and therefore equals male. Within this traditional view of health care as a male domain, the concept of health itself is also male defined. Despite the fact that women provide the bulk of the health labour force, they are neither seen as health care providers nor recognised as powerful within the health care system. Game (1983) suggests that the division of labour in health care is the most blatant form of sexual polarisation, with male medicine dominating the other predominantly female health professions.

Although medicine is still perceived as a traditionally male profession, women are entering medical schools in increasing numbers. Current admission rates to the University of New South Wales Faculty of Medicine run at 50 per cent for women. In her article on women in health care occupations, Wyndham (1983) explodes some of the myths surrounding women in medicine. The first of these is that women doctors have a higher drop out rate and the second is that they work fewer hours per week and fewer years per lifetime. Although erroneous, these arguments still persist and are used to substantiate the often made claim cited by both Fett (1976) and Wyndham that educating women to become doctors is not as good an investment as educating men.

However, although in Australia and similar countries more women are entering the medical profession, they are still under-represented in senior academic and administrative positions and in the specialties, and over-represented in part time, low paid and low status jobs. For example, the only female professors in the clinical schools in medical faculties in Australia are in Psychiatry and Community Medicine,

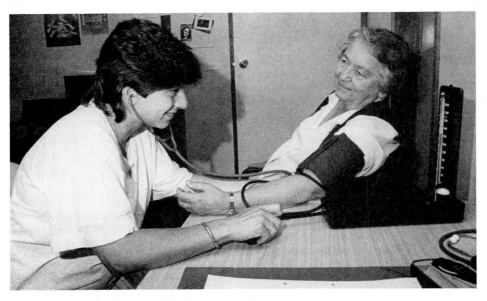

Most women doctors choose or default into general practice

and even then there are only three altogether. As Wyndham (1983) points out, it would be reasonable to assume that women would be well represented in obstetrics and gynaecology, for example. However, only approximately 8 per cent of Australian obstetricians/gynaecologists are women, with similar percentages in the USA and UK. Gordon (1989) cites 'statistics' compiled by McBride which reveal current proportions of women in postgraduate training in obstetrics and gynaecology at 29 per cent and at 34 per cent in dermatology.

Reasons cited by Saltman (1989) for this paucity of women in postgraduate training are many and include length of training, lack of role models, heavy duty schedule involving long, irregular hours, a large surgical component and discrimination against women for specialty training positions in hospitals.

Fett (1976) in her definitive study *The future of women in Australian medicine* concluded that:

in the 1970s the woman medical graduate who bears two children within five years of graduation will see them both into school by the age of 32 or earlier, and will have some 32 or more years of active life ahead.

Dennerstein (1989) in her survey of women graduates from the University of Melbourne, extends those assumptions into the 1980s. She concludes that:

very few women give up medical practice (95% women compared with 97.5% of men aged less than 60 years were still in active medical practice); women tended to work as employees while men were more often in their own private practices; gender was the single biggest predictor of income level (women earn substantially less than men); women were significantly less likely to achieve senior positions; and, women had more career interruptions than men.

Dennerstein attributes these findings rather simplistically to individual conflicts between career and family. She asserts that women were 'clearly distracted by family commitments while men gave precedence to financial matters'.

A study by Saltman (1989) of the general practice workforce reveals that the proportion of females in general practice in Australia is 20 per cent. There are no formally recognised flexible or retraining options for women to attain registerable postgraduate medical qualifications. Therefore, most women medical graduates choose, or default into general practice training where part time options are difficult but not impossible.

Political and consumer expedients which serve to change the status of women in medical practice are more often found in day-to-day general practice. Both the *National women's health policy* (1989) and the *New South Wales women's health review committee* report assert that women patients in increasing numbers are

Dr Liz

Dr Liz finds a lot of satisfaction in being a partner in general practice, but it means investing time. She works 40 hours in practice, sharing her evening and weekend rosters with eight partners in a group practice in a middle-class suburb of Melbourne.

The practice provides a large number of services and the partners own the specialist centre adjacent to the clinic. They refer patients to the centre, but also have their own theatre for minor surgery on lumps and bumps, stitching up factory workers, dental anaesthesia, IUDs and pap smears and plastering for minor breaks. There is also a small laboratory for test analysis.

It may be the medicine of the future, the general practitioner who provides a broad level of services for what doctors are calling 'the whole person'.

Says Dr Liz: 'I'm interested in the resolution of family and work problems, in the person in his or her setting whether it is marriage or a group, work relationships and interests. I enjoy it when patients see you as having the skills required to help them solve their problems.'

She has worked in 10 countries, in general practice and health planning in developed and developing countries. She is interested in illness prevention, health promotion and women's health. 'I have to be, because so many women come to women doctors. Probably under a quarter of GPs in Victoria are women'.

Her prescription for what makes a good doctor:

1. A person who is willing to update through continuing education schemes such as the family medicine program run by the College of GPs.
2. Someone who is interested in the details of a person's life and relationships, work and family, so a patient is not just a body.
3. A person who keeps up with allied health professionals and community self-help groups as well as specialists for referrals.
4. Someone who cares for his or her own family.
5. A person who is willing to work in a team.
6. Someone who is able to cope with emergencies, because the GP has a special set of skills, knowledge and attitudes.

She has little time for people with negative views about a GP's role or abilities. 'If a GP sees himself as someone on the bottom rung instead of the edge of a revolution in health care, then he has a limited vision of his role.'

The Bulletin, 21 February 1989

choosing to see women general practitioners, and not just for gynaecological consultations. As the majority of general practice patients are women, practices are recognising the market implications. The tables are turning. Male general practitioners are approaching women general practitioners to work for them and solve their 'women's problems'. This trend has not yet been recognised in the specialty areas of medicine.

Nursing

Euripides (428 BC) said that it is better to be sick than to attend to the sick. The one is a simple ill; the other combines pain of mind and toil of body.

Nurses are a major occupational group within the Australian health care system. Wyndham (1978) notes that nurses constitute 64.7 per cent of the total health workforce and 94.3 per cent of nurses are women. Eglington (1985) suggests that until recently Australian nursing has not followed the pathway of autonomous practice envisaged by Nightingale. Rather, it has created for women a sphere of paid labour in which the role of women as domestic, unpaid labourers is emulated. She goes on to conclude that the 'naturalness' of women to do the nurturing and caring tasks of nursing only serves to entrench them still deeper in the sexual division of labour in the health care workforce.

It is only recently that nurses have begun to see nursing education and practice as a profession. Eglington (1985) believes that the changes are in part due to a growing trade union consciousness. Traditionally, nurses have not been encouraged to use skills outside of health care. *The Lamp* (1985) quotes the President of the Australian Trained Nurses Association who in 1947 stated 'I have never liked trade unionism as applied to nursing'.

Long before they developed an interest in formalising their professional objectives, nurses had a well organised industrial body in New South Wales, called the NSW Nurses Association. In trade union terms, it is a small to moderately sized union. In 1981 the membership of this union consisted of approximately:

- 1500 members in the Principles and Practices Division (nurse educators and directors of nursing);
- 5000 members in the Crown Division (psychiatric nurses); and
- 25000 members in the General Division.

In the second half of the 1980s the three divisions were amalgamated.

The principal nursing trade union in the rest of Australia, except for Queensland, is the Royal Australian Nursing Federation. In 1988 the Federation amalgamated with the NSW Nurses Association. The major issues concerning nurses over the last ten years have been wages, working hours and the establishment of a career structure. Each of these issues has resulted in some form of industrial action being taken by nurses. Despite an amalgamated union, wages and conditions vary from state to state, e.g. following industrial action in NSW, a 38 hour week for nurses with a ten hour break between shifts was achieved.

Although nursing was just like a trade with a trade union, nurses did not use the 'ultimate' industrial action weapon — the strike — until 1979. This was prompted by government cuts to health spending. During the strike, patient safety was ensured by maintaining a skeleton staff. It is interesting to note that nurses have not taken strike action over their own wages and conditions, but rather over employer decisions affecting numbers of jobs and health facilities. As the Australian newspaper, *The Age* (1985), pointed out: 'the government must be aware that the Florence Nightingale factor can no longer be relied upon to keep nurses at work during industrial disputes.' As a direct result of these strikes the federal government implemented a taskforce to look into the recruitment situation and to make recommendations.

Over the last ten years of industrial action, nurses membership of unions has increased fourfold. Gray (1984) established a strong correlation between job satisfaction and attitudinal militancy. She suggested several predisposing sociological conflicts:

- the overwhelming predominance of women in this occupation;
- the implied subservience of an altruistic orientation;
- the changing attitude of women to their work and roles in society; and
- the changing nature of the hospital hierarchy.

Gray's studies have shown that student nurses are more militant than registered nurses. Griffin (1981) disputes this assertion.

An editorial in *The Lamp* (1984) quotes a 1982 Australia-wide study of nurses' political participation. Nurses were asked whether they were as politically active outside their employing institutions as they should be. 'No' was the answer received from 88 per cent of respondents.

The major reasons given for this negative response included:

- nurses' socialisation;
- apathy;
- lack of motivation; and
- the belief that nursing should not be political.

It was apparent that at that time nurses did not perceive themselves as part of a cohesive group. There appeared to be no sense of shared belonging or identification of sharing similar problems and situations.

As previously pointed out, a profession involves advanced education. Educational objectives are important in defining the area of expertise to which the profession is laying claim. Nursing training has now moved out of the hospitals, where trainee nurses traditionally provided a cheap labour supply, and into the undergraduate and postgraduate curricula of universities. However, full recognition of nursing is slow. The availability of degree courses in nursing in Australia is not universal (Russell 1990).

In recognising that women's working life is substantially different to that of men's, the taskforce recommended primary changes in the areas of conditions of employment and improvements in the workplace. One major change was the recognition that many women would be able to return to the nursing profession if part time and job share positions were introduced. Hospital administrations had previously not generally accepted part time or casual placements as feasible work options. According to Game (1982), hospital administrations were concerned that

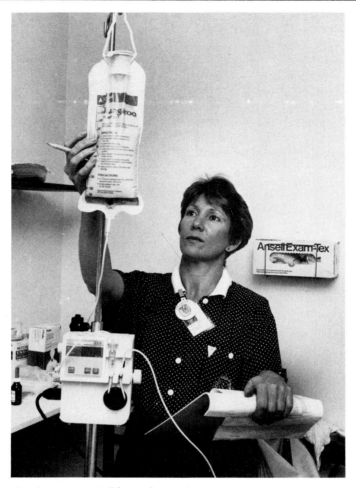

Nursing education is now essential for professional practice

part time nurses might disrupt full time ones because of their more favourable job conditions. It was also a concern for the nurses, as part timers might 'pick the eyes' out of the shifts, leaving the least favourable to full timers. As a consequence, full time and part time nurses tend to be employed in separate areas.

The taskforce also recognised that child care facilities were essential in encouraging women to return to nursing. The report highlighted the difficulties women experienced in combining their professional and domestic responsibilities. Long hours, rotating rosters and short breaks between shifts were a continuing source of exasperation and stress.

In terms of education and training, the taskforce recommended refresher courses to encourage trained nurses to return to the profession. It also recommended that the move from hospital based education to college based education be examined and strategies developed to cope with the inadequate numbers of nurse graduates in 1987 or subsequent years. These findings were published in *The Lamp* (1987).

In their struggle to gain comparative wages and conditions and recognition of skills, nurses have achieved considerable gains. However, it is predicted that, with increased college based education, nurses will become more militant in seeking greater control over their workplace and recognition at the decision making and policy levels. The masculinisation of the profession may also expedite this process. Changes in nursing began to accelerate as men entered its ranks. Today, there is a disproportionately large number of men in positions of power within the nursing profession. Eglington (1989) believes this has two implications. Firstly, the increasing numbers of men entering the profession ensures that legitimisation of nursing as a profession will proceed quickly. Secondly, the models of career development established in male dominated professions will permeate nursing and facilitate fast career advancement for these men.

Other health professions

Other members of the health care team include: physiotherapists, occupational therapists and social workers. Like nursing, these areas have traditionally been predominantly female. As such, they are open to all the criticisms levelled at feminine occupations, including 'wastage' of training when women break from their careers, often for child rearing purposes, a supposed lack of career commitment and a relatively young work force. It has been suggested that these women are merely filling in time before Mr Right, or preferably Dr Right, comes along.

Consider the case of occupational therapy. Current research indicates that significant numbers of qualified occupational therapists will have left the full time workforce by the time they are 30. According to the National Survey of the Occupational Therapy Labour Force (1981) cited by Griffin (1985), only 25 per cent of practising occupational therapists planned to continue more than 10 years in the profession from the time of survey. Of those practising (75 per cent of the survey population) over half (53 per cent) were under 30 years of age with only 11 per cent over 45 years of age. Griffin (1985) quotes Taylor's study (1983) citing that the majority of those not practicising had left the profession before turning 30 years of age and three out of every four had been away from the profession for up to six years.

Women are still predominantly held responsible for child rearing tasks and only 5 per cent of the surveyed institutions provided child care facilities for staff. In addition, part time jobs and job sharing arrangements are difficult to find.

In spite of their lower status, research indicates that students training in the ancillary professions do not see themselves as handmaidens. Surveys of students in occupational therapy, speech therapy and physiotherapy at Cumberland College of Health Sciences cited by Griffin (1985) suggest that paramedical students are autonomous both in their ideas and behaviour. These students exhibit low levels of deference and abasement. They do not always want to conform and do what is expected. Their higher aggression shows a willingness to criticise other points of view and to express anger. Clarke and White (1983) supported this view in their findings that occupational therapists have high achievement motivation.

Mary Collins (1987) argues a similar new militancy for physiotherapists:

Over the past decade there have been very significant changes in medical technology, the needs of the community, the health care workforce and the economy. These same forces have created a need to develop the physiotherapy profession: its skill and knowledge base, its role and contribution, its own identity and its image in health and community contexts. This change requires that we develop ourselves collectively in order to maintain our relevance and effectiveness in the light of our increased understanding of women's health issues and their needs as clients. As we change our knowledge, skills and identity, we can begin to contribute in new and more effective ways. Similarly, as we change our image in the eyes of other health care professionals and the community, they are more likely to call on us to make new and more effective contributions.

Short and Eglington (1987) assert that physiotherapy has traditionally attracted three types of women:

- women of independent means, including girls in training or those girls 'marking time before marriage and family';
- working mothers, including those women with family responsibilities; and
- career women, including women who have played leading roles in the profession.

The Physiotherapists' Registration Board of NSW in its manpower survey of 1983 found that nearly one-third of registered physiotherapists are currently not practising. Of the remaining two-thirds, one-third are in private practice. Short and Eglington (1987) believe that the physiotherapy 'wastage' is in part due to the working conditions and the subservient attitudes expected of physiotherapists.

The sexual division of labour in health care is not a uniquely Australian problem. In 1982 the Health Manpower division of the World Health Organization carried out a multinational study of women as providers of health. Their findings were similar to those in Australian studies: that women held less prestigious and lower paid jobs than men for several reasons including:

- a lower general standard of education;
- specific recruitment of women into lower paid positions;
- the dual responsibilities of family and work;
- lack of leadership training; and
- lack of continuing training and employment structures which did not cater to women's needs.

Privatisation

Privatisation of health care services, especially domestic services in hospitals, is a growing trend in the northern hemisphere. Several attempts have been made in Australia to introduce contract services into government run health care. The private sector does not have a good track record in providing a working environment conducive to women. Privatisation and contracting of work will hit women in the workforce hardest. Salaried staff, mainly women, will have no voice in this private notion of health care, and they stand to lose their government jobs, which include the small gains women have won in their working environment, e.g.

holidays, superannuation, sick pay, and maternity leave. The privatisation of this area of health care has already occurred in the UK. Contractors are usually companies, still a male domain. Although these women may be re-employed by contractors, the lessons learnt from other women working as casuals in the community, e.g. cleaners and garment industry outworkers are ominous.

Unpaid women workers in health care

A group of women health care workers who are substantial in number yet almost invisible are the women who look after the health of their families. Traditionally it has been the role of women to be the primary health carers in the home. Mothers have always been in charge of the medicine chest: diagnosing, prescribing and dispensing. Whilst this role has primarily been directed to the emerging, younger family, it is now also directed to the declining, older family. Daughters are often in charge of the home health care of their elderly parents. Braithwaite (1986) and Gibson (1984) have studied the unpaid health care workforce in Australia. Both studies found that women were the major health care providers for their families, particularly the older members of the family. As nurses are the handmaidens of doctors, mothers, wives and daughters are the handmaidens of households and look after health care aspects at home. Braithwaite has also suggested that the women who provide these unpaid services encounter great difficulties — they are at best, unrecognised as legitimate health care providers and, at worst, unsupported (see table 5.1).

WOMEN AS CONSUMERS OF HEALTH CARE

The role, user of health care services, has been given various titles within the health care professions. The medical title is 'patient'. However, this term is too limiting as it refers to an illness/disease model of health care. Critics of this term would also suggest that 'patient' implies a deferential power dynamic with the medical profession. Other health care providers e.g. nurses and social workers choose to refer to the woman as a 'client'. This term, it is believed is less value laden and more accurately reflects both a satisfactory power relationship and appropriate expectations of both parties. Client does however have a financial implication. It assumes that the service is attracting a financial reimbursement. As was argued earlier in this chapter and will be argued in others, privatisation of health care in any form disadvantages women. Women generally have lower socio-economic status than their male counterparts and therefore are often unable to buy any, let alone the best, health care. The term 'consumer' avoids the financial implications and links women in the health care system to the emerging powerful consumers' movement. Unfortunately, this word also has its limitations. It implies that health care is a consumable item. Often the definition of what is actually 'consumed' is problematic. However, the notion of using up finite resources is also implied in this term. In an ever-shrinking health economy, this is a useful framework to maintain. Therefore, whilst no term is perfect, this book will use consumer to describe the non-provider role in health care.

Women and sickness

There are many myths surrounding the subject of women and sickness. Women are sicker than men but men die younger. How can this apparent contradiction in terms be true?

One reason why women live longer than men is that oestrogen gives them a biological advantage. However, until this century, perinatal and maternal mortality during childbirth completely annulled this advantage. Women died in childbirth and, in some cultures, if a choice had to be made between saving the life of the mother or the child, certain religious imperatives demanded the child be spared. Also, attempts were more likely to be made to save male newborn.

This biological advantage is still maintained despite significant social disadvantage. However, this edge may once again be neutralised when the feminisation

Table 5.1: Changes in carer's lifestyle since caring began

Changes in lifestyle	No. of carers responding	Carers mentioning %				Total
		Improvement	No change	Deterioration	Not applicable	
Time available for leisure/recreation	1561	4.5	26.9	67.9	0.6	100
Family's financial situation	155	7.7	69.7	18.1	4.5	100
Performance at work	155	2.6	25.2	7.1	65.2	100
Plans for job-seeking	156	3.2	30.1	11.5	55.1	100
Ability to get housework done	156	3.8	44.2	49.4	2.6	100
Own health and stamina	157	5.1	38.9	55.4	0.6	100
Relationship with spouse	155	3.9	41.3	17.4	37.4	100
Relationship with own children	157	9.5	47.8	17.8	24.8	100
Relationship with siblings	157	6.4	52.2	21.7	19.7	100
How carer got along with elderly relative	157	14.6	56.7	28.7	-	100
How close carer felt to elderly relative	156	21.1	59.0	19.2	0.6	100
Relationship with friends	157	7.6	55.4	33.8	3.2	100
General emotional state	156	5.8	35.3	59.0	-	100
Feelings about self	155	12.3	57.4	29.0	1.3	100
Ability to relax/sleep through night	157	7.6	36.3	56.1	-	100
Feelings about growing older	157	13.4	50.3	35.7	0.6	100
Plans for the future	157	10.2	48.4	23.6	17.8	100

(Rossiter, Kinnear and Graycar 1984)

of poverty is more complete. McDonald (1985) has stressed the urgent problem of women in poverty. The *National women's health policy* (1989) highlighted poverty amongst Aboriginal women as increasingly more obvious.

Another argument for why women live longer is that, by comparison, men have a sociological disadvantage. For example, they are more likely to go to war and die than women. Men are also more prone to include themselves in risk taking behaviour. Men are more successful in their attempts to commit suicide, particularly during adolescence and early adulthood (see chapter three). Men smoke more cigarettes and drink more alcohol than women. Hence the higher prevalence of smoking and drink-driving related deaths in men. However, some of this behaviour, particularly smoking and drinking is increasing amongst women.

How do we know that women are sicker than men? This raises the issue of the ways in which sickness is recorded.

One way is through hospital admissions. Women are admitted to hospital more than men. There are two reasons for this:

1. in Australia, childbirth is most often a hospital event. Nearly all deliveries are conducted in hospitals. The argument whether childbirth should be a hospital or home practice still continues. In Australia, where the Caesarean rate (operative childbirth) is high, childbirth is at best seen as risk-taking behaviour. (see chapter seven); and
2. as women live longer than men, they therefore survive to ages in which chronic illness predominates and often require hospital admission, e.g. hip fractures.

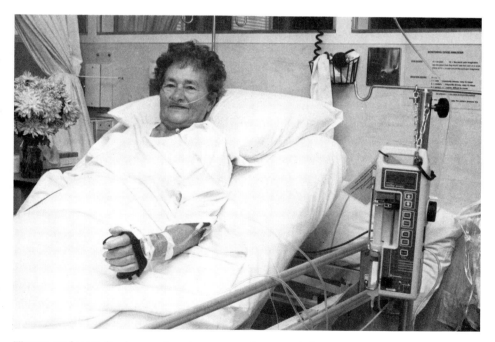

Women are hospitalised more often than men predominantly for reproductive concerns

In Australia, visiting the doctor is also more likely to be a women's event. Social acceptance of illness is higher for women. Not only do they represent the major non-paid health care provider, but also the family advocate in the local health network. Women take their children and parents to the doctor. Events in the life cycle of women are also labelled as medical events, e.g. reproduction. Women may attend health care services when perfectly well for either contraceptive advice or preventive screening for cancers of the reproductive system. Ironically preventive consultations, such as those mentioned, are recorded under an illness framework.

Certain life events, such as reproduction and prevention of illness, e.g. Pap smears, are erroneously labelled as sickness. This means women are more likely to be erroneously labelled as sick than men, when experiencing certain natural responses (see chapter nine). For example, men are depressed, women suffer from depression; menopause is an endocrine deficiency disorder, not a natural process of ageing.

Sickness certification is another form of record keeping that can serve to label women as sick. In the workforce, a sickness certificate legitimises work absence for both worker and employer. It may be the only way a working woman can legitimately take time off to seek medical attention for a sick child, disabled relative or elderly parent. In this way, work absences are inappropriate measures of sickness for women.

Alternatives to conventional health care

It is no wonder that women are becoming more angry and frustrated with conventional health care systems. In consultation meetings with Liza Newby, who formulated the *National women's health policy*, women were 'very enthusiastic about the concept of special women's health centres because of:

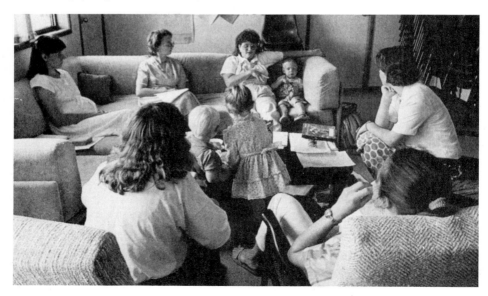

A postnatal support group at a women's health centre in Wollongong

- no or minimum charges;
- the possibility of multidisciplinary services in one location;
- a holistic approach to care;
- the availability of prevention information and advice;
- health promotion activities; and
- participation in decisions about their own care'.

Since the turn of the century, women have been involved in the provision of health care services that were specifically for women, albeit in the area of reproductive health, e.g. the forerunner of the Queen Victoria Hospital in Adelaide was essentially planned by a group of women. During the 1970s, the focus shifted from reproduction to fertility control, as the Family Planning Association took shape.

Women's health centres were established in Australia initially to provide services for women in areas where they were not receiving adequate service in conventional health care institutions. Reproduction is not the only health need addressed by these centres. Since their inception they have expanded their brief beyond service provision to become centres of consumer education and networking. They are staffed and run by women's collectives. Women's refuges and rape crisis centres are further developments. Unfortunately, their funding by both state and federal government grants, is always in jeopardy. It has been suggested that the almost regular reviews of women's health services in Australia is a mechanism designed to tire women to the point where they cease to ask for their needs to be met or have any expectations.

Whilst women's health centres allow women the opportunity to regain control over their own bodies, other strategies are also used to achieve this goal. Two further approaches have achieved popularity in the process of addressing the issues of paternalism and lack of accurate information.

One approach addresses the question of women educating themselves about health. This process has occurred in both formal and informal ways. In the long term, strategies have been directed to enable structural change in the way women see their health. Examples of this include:

- in secondary schools girls are learning about their health in personal development and/or health classes;
- in the academic environment, Women and health courses have been established for many years in Women's studies and Community Health programs, e.g. at the University of New South Wales; and
- more recently, formal programs have been established in nursing curricula and a Key Centre for Women's Health has been established at the University of Melbourne.

More practical strategies have been employed to address the present problems of women in the community. The development of a women-centred health consumers forum and resource information networks have aided women in developing programs to allow them to collect, understand and evaluate health information in appropriate ways. *Our Bodies, Ourselves* the North American consumer 'textbook' on women and health is the result of such groups of women identifying key health issues of women and recording women friendly information.

Information may not only be textbook. Women's life experiences provide most valuable information on health care, particularly on the natural course of illness, chronic illness and reproductive health. Groups of women networking to discuss common health themes have been the basis of the self-help and self-care movements both in Australia and the United States.

Exploration of other forms of health care is another approach. There is a tendency for people to label this type of health care 'alternative'. Unfortunately, the term 'alternative' is misleading, as it implies a lesser, or second string approach, in the same way that 'ancillary' implies an inferior status. Conventional health care has had, and probably always will have, huge gaps in the services it can provide. This is particularly true in the areas of chronic illness and reproductive health. Some options include:

- acupuncture;
- chiropractic;
- homeopathy;
- iridology;
- massage;
- meditation and relaxation;
- creative movement;
- art and music therapy etc.

It is beyond the scope of this book to explore these other forms of health care.

CASE STUDY: ONE

Nicholas is a dark eyed, black haired, two year old who lives in a suburban home with his parents and an older brother and an older sister.

Recently he spent a night in hospital.

Nicholas was his usual bouncy, babbling self in the morning, but his mother noticed that he did not eat all of his lunch, and he had a longer sleep than usual in the afternoon. By dinner time he was hot, not interested in eating and had developed a cough. By 4 a.m. he was having difficultly breathing and his parents took him to the nearby children's hospital. He was seen quickly by a nurse and then a doctor because he was obviously in a lot of discomfort, and the noise of his laboured breathing was alarming. He was given an injection — his parents were not sure what that was for — and his breathing improved after he began to use a humidifier. It was a long and anxious couple of hours. Nicholas's mother remained with him on her own, while her husband took the other children home to sleep. They had come into the hospital, but were tired and fractious and had become querulous, disturbing the other patients and staff. The paediatrician on duty complimented Nicholas's mother on their decision to bring him to hospital that night because his condition could have become serious quite rapidly. He then asked her whether she wanted to take her son home, or have him admitted to hospital. She was shocked. She had just begun to relax a little. 'For heaven's sake! What kind of a question is that? Isn't that the doctor's decision to make? You decide, not me!'

The doctor suggested they sit down while he explained about Nicholas's problem. But his mother's mind was questioning 'Is he incompetent? Why does he ask me what I want? I'm only the baby's mother!'

CASE STUDY: TWO

Clare was early arriving at her office in the new primary health care centre this morning because the sudden cold snap at the beginning of winter might mean several extra patients to call on. Clare is responsible for community occupational therapy in a rural township and the farmlands surrounding it. Part of a river valley the area is a grazing and farming community with many small supportive light industries too. These have grown up because the area is eight hours driving time from the State capital, and four hours to the regional centre.

Much of the work of the community health team involves assisting elderly people who have retired into the township.

Accident rehabilitation is time consuming too, and the team has launched an accident awareness program because of an increasing number of hand injuries associated with accidents in the manufacturing machinery and repair plants.

Clare attended to the forms and messages in her office first: the results of the pilot study for the accident awareness programme were pleasing, and the proofs of the new poster campaign are ready for viewing. Mary Clarke is worried about her son's progress at his new school — his burn scars are still very visible. Mrs Lineman needs a new shower seat.

It was then time to start her calls. Her first visit was to Beryl, an elderly women who had run a cafe-restaurant in the town for thirty years, but who had recently retired because her arthritis was causing her too much pain and prevented her enjoying the job she used to love. Beryl had run the petrol station part of the business too in the twenty years since her husband had died, and now was happy to hand all of it over to her daughter Sandra. It suited Sandra too, because at forty five her youngest child was fifteen, and she was looking for a challenge and new activities in her life. Of course Sandra was airing a few ideas that Beryl didn't exactly agree with, but she liked the idea of still doing her bit by helping with the cooking for the family, and filling in at the cafe if they were particularly busy. Of course Beryl knew everything that was happening in town as almost everyone visited her regularly. That was one thing she was finding very hard to accept, she had always been at the centre of things, and now she was on the outside and felt resentful and lonely much of the time.

When Clare arrived Beryl was feeling quite sorry for herself; the cold weather was making her hips and knees ache dreadfully, and several of her friends had not made the trip into town because of the weather. They were pleased to see each other — Beryl liked to hear from Clare how her friends were, and for Clare at the beginning of a long day, Beryl's coffee and down to earth humour were somehow reassuring and encouraging. Clare delivered the rails and other aids which were to be installed in Beryl's bathroom, and told her she had arranged with an electrician to change some of the switches and plugs in her house to make them easier to use with her painful and stiff fingers.

Next Clare checked on Joel who had been a paraplegic since a car accident eight years previously. Joel conducted his own accountancy business from home, but had been having a bit of trouble lately with bladder infections and Clare was helping him change his working timetable somewhat.

Today he was angry and tired; every now and again things got him down and today was one of those days. So instead of making suggestions about his work timetable, they just chatted for a while. He found that it often helped to share his frustrations with someone like Clare who really did understand his difficulties. Later in the week they would talk about work.

After visiting an elderly woman who was recovering from a stroke and needing advice about preparing food, Clare decided to stop for lunch.

Somehow the days went by like this — one after the other, very routine. As she drove along she wondered what she was REALLY doing. Did her work actually make anyone healthier or happier, or better able to cope with their lives and their illnesses...?

REFERENCES

Alford, R.A. (1972). The political economy of health care: dynamics without change, *Politics and society*, 2, 127–164.

Braithwaite, V. (1986). The burden of home care: how is it shared? *In Supplement to Community health studies*, X, 3, NH & MRC Social Psychiatry Research Unit, ANU, Canberra.

Collins, M. (1987). *Women's health through lifestages — the physiotherapist's contribution*, Australian Physiotherapy Association (NSW Branch).

Dennerstein, L. (1989). Survey finds women's medical careers still constrained, *Australian medicine*, 1, 423.

Eglington, E.A. (1985). *Australian trade unions: why have NSW nurses become more militant?* paper presented to the 2nd national conference of The Women Workers in Health Care Association.

Eglington, E.A. (1989). *The nursing workforce*, WHO conference proceedings, inter country workshop on primary health care, China.

Fett, I. (1976). The future of women in Australian medicine, *The medical journal of Australia*, 2, 33–39.

Furler, E. (1985). Women and health: radical prevention, *New doctor*, 37, 5–8.

Game, A. & Pringle, R. (1982). *Gender at work*, Allen & Unwin, Sydney.

Gibson, R. (1984). Community vs. institutional care: the case of the Australian aged, *Journal of social science in medicine*, 18, 997–1004.

Gordon, G. (1989). Women in post-graduate training, *Australian medicine*, 1, 423.

Gray, D. (1984). Attitudinal militancy amongst Australian nurses, *Australian journal of social issues*, 19, 2.

Griffin, G. (1981). Personal characteristics and industrial militancy in white collar unions, *Journal of industrial relations*, 23, 2.

Griffin, S. (1985). *Occupational therapy: a female profession*, UNSW Masters thesis.

McDonald, P. (1985). *The economic consequences of marriage breakdown in Australia: a summary*, Australian institute of family studies, Melbourne.

National Women's Health Policy (1989). *National women's health policy: advancing women's health in Australia*, AGPS, Canberra.

Rossiter, C., Kinnear, D. & Graycar, A. (1984). *Family care of elderly people: 1983 survey results*, Social Welfare Research Centre Reports and Proceedings, no. 38, January.

Russell, L.R. (1990). *From nightingale to now: nurse education in Australia*, W.B. Saunders, Sydney.

Saltman, D.C. (1989). Medicine: a textbook on discrimination, *Australian doctor*, October, 113.

Short, S. & Eglington, E.A. (1987). *Militancy in nursing and physiotherapy*, paper presented to the 2nd national conference of The women workers in health care association.

The Age (1985). 22 Oct.

The Lamp (1984). March 17.

The Lamp (1987). October 4.

The Lamp (1985). April 15.

WHO (1983). *1982 Health Manpower Study*, WHO Chronicle, Geneva.

Wyndham, D. (1983). Women in health occupations: prospects for doctors and other health workers, *Healthright*, 2, 22–27.

6 Women and Sexuality

A woman's sexuality comprises the sum of her knowledge, beliefs and attitudes, and predicts the way she will behave with regard to her sexual activity. It is subject to lifelong dynamic changes. Sexuality has three components: biological, social, and psychological. De Beauvoir (1972) reflected the growing awareness of women about their bodies and their sexual self in her comment 'it is not nature that defines woman; it is she who defines herself by dealing with nature on her own account'. It was not until the 1970s that women centred literature on sexuality emerged. The Boston Women's Health Book Collective (1978), the Hite report (1976) and the work of Sheila Kitzinger (1983) all demonstrate the broad context of women's sexuality which involves their sexual responsiveness, sexual expression and sexual needs.

BIOLOGICAL DETERMINISM: THE CASE FOR WOMEN AND ANIMALS

Much energy has been directed into defining the biological components of reproduction (see chapter 7). As information about the reproductive process becomes more technical, the tendency to define sexuality in reproductive terms increases. Koutroulis (1990) asserts that the medical profession, and in particular obstetricians and gynaecologists, reinforce biological determinism as a major component of women's sexuality. Such scientific endeavour often results in a restrictive definition of women rather than enabling them to develop. For example Yerkes'

Female sexuality between the lines

The emergence of the women's health movement in Australia in the past decade has provided abundant evidence that women are far from satisfied with the quality of their heath care and the way it is delivered.

Women have complained that they have different health needs to men that are not being met sensitively or effectively. The tone of these complaints was captured in a report three years ago by the women's health policy working party in Victoria, in which many women described doctors as sexist, moralistic and intimidating.

Sexist attitudes among doctors may reflect the values of society at large, but a study by a Melbourne researcher suggests that doctors' medical education may also shape these attitudes. The researcher, Glenda Koutroulis, analysed gynaecology and obstetric textbooks used in Australian medical schools and found they were pervaded by 'a hidden curriculum of sexist, patriarchal ideology' often masquerading as science.

Ms Koutroulis, a member of the health sociology research group at La Trobe University and a nurse educator, says the texts implied that women were expected to reproduce, to have reason clouded by their emotions, to be passive, dependent, seductive, manipulative and untrustworthy.

The study followed the path carved 17 years ago in the United States by Diana Scully and Pauline Bart, whose paper in *The American Journal of Sociology* was entitled 'A Funny Thing Happened On The Way To The Orifice: Women In Gynaecology Textbooks'.

Scully and Bart were interested in the extent to which the findings of experts on human sexuality were reflected in the textbooks. They said that in 1953, when Kinsey and associates published 'Sexual Behaviour in the Human Female', doctors for the first time had authoritative information on female sexuality.

Although Kinsey debunked the Freudian dictum that vaginal orgasm was the only mature sexual response, gynaecologists tenaciously clung to the idea. Scully and Bart said that, as late as 1965, gynaecology texts were reporting the vagina as the main erogenous zone.

While most of the 15 books analysed by Glenda Koutroulis did not contain outdated and incorrect information about women's sexual response, the sexist ideology was still there. Women's sexuality was still depicted from a heterosexual perspective, with marriage and mothering the 'natural' aspirations of all women.

The books were on the recommended reading lists at Melbourne, Monash, Flinders and Newcastle universities. Two of the texts were co-authored by women, but Ms Koutroulis says there was no discernible difference between these and the others in the way women were portrayed.

She found that female sexuality was virtually ignored in the books, although when it was discussed there was a vast improvement in the way the Australian texts reflected current information. There was little mention of 'frigidity', a term that Scully and Bart had found repeatedly. The books no longer presented sex as primarily for reproduction, or considered that the male sex drive was stronger than the female's.

It was hoped that such studies would bring improvements. At first glance, Ms Koutroulis says, it appears the authors of *Illustrated Textbook of Gynaecology* have seen the importance of findings such as those of Scully and Bart, to women. The authors wrote: 'Dissatisfaction has been expressed loudly by activist groups against authoritarianism, paternalism, insensitivity, sexist attitudes, and disease orientation rather than patient orientation ... This has sometimes extended to the formation of clinics run by women themselves who have been unable to find their Dr Kindheart and Dr Takecare.'

Glenda Koutroulis says this last condescending comment undermines all that was previously said, suggesting that the authors were unconvinced by the seriousness of what they had just presented.

Ms Koutroulis found a number of recurring themes. For example, on women and the child-rearing role, women were held almost entirely responsible for the ills of their offspring and family, she says. 'The assumption is that women are not only the prime child-rearers, but the only child-rearers, as the role of men is ignored.'

Another theme was marital obsession. Ms Koutroulis says women's marital and sexual status were defined through their relationships with men; the texts assumed most women were married.

There was also a concern with women's marital performance. Discussing marital dysfunction during a woman's child-bearing years, the authors of *Illustrated Textbook of Gynaecology* state 'in some instances the breakdown will be related to the superwoman syndrome — the mother who struggles to keep her career, home and enlarging family under control'.

Implicitly, this was too much for her and there was something wrong with doing it, Ms Koutroulis says. If she did do it, she became responsible for marital breakdown. 'Biological determinism is the hidden curriculum of this statement which can be more clearly seen if we change the gender so that it reads: 'In some instances the breakdown will be related to the superman syndrome — the father who struggles to keep his career, home and enlarging family under control.'

The textbooks also contained a persistent, outdated preoccupation with women as virgins. A photograph in *Color Atlas of Gynaecology* carries the caption: Coital laceration of the vagina in a single, 28-year-old woman. She was not virginal, but experienced severe deep pain during savage intercourse with a casual acquaintance during a visit by ship to Melbourne.' Ms Koutroulis says the references to the women's marital and sexual status are irrelevant.

She found that gynaecologists commented on the psyche as well as the reproductive tract of women, in some cases inappropriately suggesting a psychiatric basis for certain behaviour. For example, post-birth reactions of women, such as insomnia, come under suspicion as psychiatrically induced, when the causes may be social or normal.

And while in *Gynaecology Illustrated* a woman who described menstrual pain as 'a red hot drill' was labelled neurotic, Ms Koutroulis says that from her experience no such label is applied to a man who says of prostrate pain 'It feels like I'm pissing nails'.

Glenda Koutroulis argues that by presenting opinion and prejudice under the guise of objective science, the textbooks do not provide medical students with an appropriate model of women. Nor were the books sympathetic to the ideals of treatment that women had consistently expressed a desire for.

The authors of gynaecology and obstetric textbooks are by no means the only ones liable to criticism. A Melbourne doctor who lectures in women's health said that *Anatomy: Regional and Applied*, the main anatomy text for undergraduates and surgical trainees shows a diagram of the female pelvis in which some areas appear empty. She says these spaces are not in fact empty, but contain erectile tissue which is known to exist.

Glenda Koutroulis argues that an urgent review of educational material on women's health and sexuality is needed. Unfortunately, she believes an increase in the number of female medical students offers no guarantee of an improvement in doctors' attitudes towards women.

'Indeed the reverse may happen as women doctors strive to be accepted in a profession entrenched in a male-dominated perspective,' she says. 'Such pressure could result in women doctors accepting the traditional ways of practice and behaviour and turning away from the cries of a few.'

Philip McIntosh, *The Age*, 11 July 1990

(1943) work on chimpanzees' reproductive functions makes cultural assumptions about females:

When the female (chimpanzee) is not sexually receptive the naturally more dominant member of the pair almost regularly obtains the food; whereas during the female's phase of maximum genital swelling, when she is sexually receptive, she claims or may claim the food and take it regularly even though she be the naturally subordinate member of the pair.

Herschberger (1970) in her critique of Yerkes' work separates the genital components of sexuality from the sociological argument. She poses the problem of balancing the biological and sociological components:

> It was quite a feat of nature to grant the small clitoris the same number of nerves as the penis. It was an even more incredible feat that society should actually have convinced the possessors of this organ that it was sexually inferior to the penis.

McIntosh (1978) addresses the dilemma. She cites the work of Gagnon and Simon (1974) in proposing that the sexual behaviour of women like any other behaviour is socially scripted, that is, that if women behave sexually in a particular way it is because there is a range of socially available patterns of behaviour for them to learn. Whilst she limits her discussion to western societies, McIntosh argues these scripts have confined women's sexual activities. Quadrio (1983) highlights the negative influence of sex role stereotyping on the development of women's sexuality. Women are seen as passive, dependent, other-directed, expressive, nurturant and sexually passive.

Sexual rituals of traditional cultures and animal models have been used to broaden the western view of whether women want sex and, if so, what sort. Katchadourian's (1985) dissertation on 'sexually permissive cultures' of the Polynesian Islands highlights how the western view of female sexuality can also pollute our observations of other cultures. Rather than enlarging review beyond biology, he strengthens the biological argument:

> Sex for Mangaian men and women means coitus, pure and simple. To that end, foreplay (including mouth-genital stimulation) is freely practised; 'dirty talk', music, scents, and nudity further heighten arousal. Women are active sexual partners psychologically as well as physically. Female orgasm, often multiple, is considered a necessary outcome of successful coitus; its absence is feared to be injurious to the woman's health. Pregnancy does not inhibit Mangaians, who continue to engage in sex up to the onset of labor pains. Parenthood strengthens further the sexual ties of a couple.

> But the Mangaian experience also demonstrates the constraint and contradictions that exist even in a society known for its unabashed and unrestrained celebration of sex throughout life. Much of premarital sexual activity, for instance, goes on covertly for the sake of maintaining appearances, and there is a certain ambivalence coloring the relationship of sexual partners. Unlike our culture where sex is expected to follow love, the Mangaians start with sex and hope that it will lead to affection. This tends to cast their sexual relations in a more physical and mechanistic mold.

Descriptions of sexual practices in other cultures lend support to the argument that women's sexuality is suppressed in the western culture. Sexual expectations and opportunities for women are limited by father, husband, church and state.

The theme of reproduction cannot be separated from an exploration of women's sexuality. The lack of education about contraception and the inability of medical researchers to develop failsafe contraception has ensured that the Victorian notions of sexual expression solely for the purposes of procreation have survived in the twentieth century although the Pill has changed this to a limited extent.

Financial and structural dependency of women ensured that these beliefs were not only held by men but also by women. There are many barriers for women which prevent them from exploring their sexual identity and accepting the behaviours of other women.

PSYCHOLOGICAL DESTINY: THE CASE FOR MEASURING WOMEN

The psychological approach focuses on the object choice or sexual orientation of a woman and her sexual responses. Freud was a pioneer in exploring this area. He used the case study approach to exploring women's sexuality. Freud's view of female sexuality was based on a view of masculine psychosexual behaviour as the norm and female sexuality as inferior. Masochism, envy, and narcissism, Freud believed, led the developing girl to long for a penis. Freud called this penis envy. He defined the female sexual response with the penis as the focus.

His critics have since suggested that this hostile view of women was an expression of womb envy, that is, an envy of woman's procreative ability. This argument uses biological differences to challenge the view of female inferiority. Mitchell (1974) interprets Freud's basic principles in a less biologic and more structural way. She sees his analysis of women's psycho-social development as an accurate description of the social norms for women at that time rather than an anatomical description, for example, the societal repression of women was not only reflected in their dress — tight corsets which confined the torso. Hysteria, the common woman's complaint at the time, may have been a result of a mechanical restriction to breathing, rather than psychosexual dysfunction.

Kinsey (1948) was a pioneer in the research of sexual behaviour. In the second half of this century he and Masters and Johnson continued this exploration of sexual normality within a biological framework. The female orgasm became the

Sexual liberation

The first part of the Kinsey Report, *Sexual Behaviour in the Human Male*, was published in 1948, the second, *Sexual Behaviour in the Human Female*, in 1953, presenting a monumental body of statistical research based on what 18,000 men and women said about their sex lives. But the full social effect of these studies was probably not felt until the 1960s, when the Pill provided a more reliable means of contraception than had ever existed before. Kinsey showed that there were enormous variations in sexual behaviour and that many practices that previously had been thought abnormal were perfectly normal, in the sense that many people engaged in them. Increasingly, masturbation, homosexuality and oral sex all got talked about with new openness, though with a frisson of excitement about what had been previously taboo subjects of conversation.

The sexual revolution of the 1960s would not have been possible without the contraceptive pill. It first came on the market, following its trial on Puerto Rican peasant women in 1956, as the 1960s dawned. It has been estimated that by the middle of 1966, 10 million women in different countries were on the Pill. It was the Pill that at last promised, if it did not actually provide on the spot, a separation between sex and reproduction. At last women could have intercourse without the threat of an unwanted pregnancy hanging over them.

Adapted from Sheila Kitzinger (1983), *Woman's experience of sex.*

focus of discussion on female sexuality. Performance indicators such as its presence, absence, site, intensity, potency and frequency still form the basis of current biologic exploration. Unfortunately, his own preconceived notions about innate differences between men and women overshadowed a true analysis of the sexual activity of women. Using what McIntosh (1978) calls the 'empiricist approach', Kinsey used questionnaire and observational data to confirm the socially constructed hypotheses that Ellis (1936) had proposed over a decade before. As McIntosh translates:

> The empiricist approach collates its 'data' and concludes that male sexuality is fundamentally different from female sexuality. The male sexual urge is seen as being more imperious, more spontaneous, more specifically genital in goal, but also as being aroused by objects and fantasies. The female urge is weaker, responds to approaches from a partner, is more dependent upon the entire relationship with the partner, yet the woman requires more direct physical stimulation to reach orgasm.

Herschberger (1970) believes that the cultural assumptions about basic differences between male and female, of these researchers, determined the observations they made. McIntosh confirms this belief about Kinsey and his researchers by presenting their data in a way that highlights similarities rather than differences. She concludes that:

> Instead of noting how the 'average' or typical woman differs from the average or typical man (as Kinsey highlights) we note instead how many men and women are similar. We find that there is a remarkable degree of overlap.

To enable the broadest possible view of all contributing factors, case studies are now often used by psychiatrists and psychologists as methods of scientific study of sexuality. Offir (1982) suggests that this method has many disadvantages. The woman being studied may not be typical of other people — even those in the same general socio-economic, religious or cultural group. The close relationship which develops over a long time between interviewer and woman subject may cloud findings and distort interpretation of the facts. The case study approach does however prevent the very judgmental process of overgeneralising which has plagued other forms of sexual research. Offir (1982) believes that women centred sociologists, social psychologist and cultural anthropologists can and do use the survey method to explore these issues.

It was not until the Hite Report (1976) which was concerned only with female sexuality that the broader agendas concerning the sociology and politics of sex were acknowledged. Methodologically the Hite Report has been widely criticised. However, the report breaks new ground in exploring what women like and do not like about sex. Ball (1989) suggests that women are searching for a set of basic psychological needs which when met characterise a pleasurable sexual contact. They are:

- oneness;
- intimacy;

- closeness; and
- togetherness.

This process also involves physical input from the partner of choice in the form of touching and verbal reassurance about being loved and lovable. Women need to have a feeling of well being to fully enjoy sexual experiences. Safety, in emotional, moral and contraceptive terms is often considered a necessary prerequisite.

BIOLOGY: NAMING THE PARTS

The biological element is concerned with the physical appearance of genitalia, e.g clitoris, vagina and secondary sexual organs, e.g. breasts. Recently with surgical and hormonal advances, the appearance of female sexual characteristics can be manipulated. Difficulties in adopting a baseline definition of sexuality arise in the case of male-to-female transexuals. The underlying chromosomal makeup must also form part of this baseline of female sexuality.

On a hormonal level, there has been considerable debate as to the effect of the sex hormones on sexuality and sexual response. Both men and women produce the female hormone oestrogen and the male hormone testosterone. However, the quantities of oestrogen and testosterone in males and females respectively are small. Contrary to the expected relationship between oestrogen and the female sexual response, Offir (1982) could find little work to indicate that oestrogen had any effect on a woman's desire for sex. She suggests that testosterone is a better indicator of sexual arousal in women. Sopchak and Sutherland (1960) found that women given testosterone for medical reasons sometimes show increased interest in sex. However, Hardy (1964) hypothesises that testosterone may not be a major contributor to the sexual response of women. She reasons that sexual intercourse for young women is arousal driven and that they have low testosterone levels.

Health problems link the biologic and reproductive aspects of women's sexuality. Throughout a woman's life cycle, reproductive issues can cause sexual dysfunction. Menarche, menstruation, pregnancy, abortion and menopause are all determinants in the complex equation of women's sexual responses. The menstrual cycle may determine a woman's openness to sexual response. Times of low fertility and cervical mucus impermeability, when oestrogen levels may be low together with dysmenorrhea can decrease a woman's libido. Similarly menopausal changes in the vaginal vault can make vaginal intercourse unpleasant.

Recently, sexually transmitted diseases such as chlamydia, candida, albicans, gardnerella, herpes, genitalis, human papilloma (wart) virus and human immunodeficiency virus have been added to the health concerns of sexually active women. Like the age old problems of syphilis and gonorrhea, many of these infections are asymptomatic in women and therefore go undetected. Even when these conditions are symptomatic, the social stigmata attached to women who acquire sexually transmitted diseases has also meant that these women are unlikely to seek treatment early. Many of the vaginal conditions from which women suffer, for example, atrophic vaginitis (the ageing of the vagina) and allergic vaginitis (allergy to the latex of barrier methods such as condoms and diaphragms) are not sexually transmitted. The distinction between sexually transmitted infections and vaginitis occurring for other reasons is rarely made clear to women by their health providers.

SPECIAL NEEDS: NAMING GROUPS

The *National women's health policy* (1989) reported that although sexuality was relevant for all women, four groups had identified specific issues:

- younger women;
- lesbians;
- women entering menopause; and
- disabled women.

Young women

Young women in their early adolescent years are establishing their sexual identity, at the same time that they are also thinking about careers and different relationships with their parents, other family members and peers. Sexuality is often not adequately addressed in the home or at school. Personal development courses were developed to facilitate this process in secondary schools. Parental, teacher and community concern as to who should be responsible for this education has led to the patchy implementation of these programs. The traditional explanation for this opposition has been that sex education leads to an increase in sexual activity. Collomb and Howard's (1988) work in the USA showed that young women did not agree with this concept. Rather they see their needs in the areas of interpersonal relationships and relative to emotional issues. In Australia, Richters (1984) reports that these courses are not run in all schools in Australia. Finlayson, Reynolds and Minn (1987) further highlight the Australian problem by suggesting that where

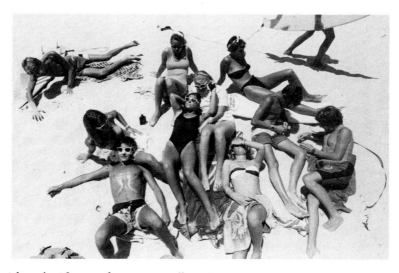

Many girls under 16 years of age are sexually active

education courses are run many of the girls view them as inappropriate. Most of the girls surveyed obtain information from their peers or from books and magazines.

The legal age of consent adds further complexity to issues of sexuality for adolescent girls. Whilst many girls under 16 years of age are sexually active, health care providers who consult with these girls and prescribe contraceptives, particularly the oral contraceptive pill, must do so with parental consent.

A woman's sense of innocence, which is a prerequisite for developing healthy sexual responsiveness in adolescence, may be lost in childhood. This loss of innocence is very relevant for incest survivors. For an incest survivor sexual experience and violation are linked. She has no experience in setting sexual limits or boundaries, in making assertive demands or in refusing sexual advances. Often the emotional attachment which is an integral part of a woman's sexual identity becomes separated. This process may also happen to adolescent girls who undergo formal initiation rites which are used in some cultures to celebrate menarche. The most widespread practice is to isolate the menstruating young girl. A Middle Eastern and African tradition of performing cliterodectomies on young girls now occurs in Australia.

Lesbians

The methods for labelling lesbians are unclear. Lockard (1986) suggests that self-identification is the only criteria by which to define lesbians. This definition would exclude at one time the vast majority of women who have questioned their sexual choice or not yet taken the difficult step of naming it. Loulan (1984) points out that, while this questioning is not only common place amongst lesbians, but also encouraged by the heterosexual community at large, no such questioning is expected in the heterosexual community of women. Queen Victoria, by not recognising female homosexuality, encapsulated society's views about lesbians. As Richards (1990) notes in her introduction to the book of *Lesbian lists*, the invisibility of the sexual act between two women and the acceptance of non sexual intimacy between two women is a continuing problem:

> how should I define a lesbian? Should I use a contemporary, twentieth-century definition? And if so, which one? Women who are sexually attracted to other women or women who become lesbians through feminism? Or should I use a much broader definition, one that includes the romantic friends movement — women who were women-identified, who had affectionate and loving relationships with other women but may not actually have had sex out of the repressive nature of the era? Should I include sworn sisters and berdaches? Should I include transvestites? Should I include spinsters?

Whilst the definition of lesbianism has been difficult, identifying alleged 'causes' has not. Homophobia, or the fear of homosexuals, both in its external forms and as lesbians internalise it, has supported a mythology of causes ranging from sexual, for example, masturbation and fear of pregnancy (1600s to early 1900s), through medical, for example, glandular imbalance (1950s), over functioning adrenal gland (1930s), cerebral abnormalities and faulty nervous organisation (1890s) and even educational, for example, women's colleges (1900s) and co-ed colleges (1900s).

As equally diverse have been the alleged 'cures' ranging from bromides, baths and bread and water in the late 19th century, to wearing dresses, separate beds, sitting on our feet and analysis in the 20th century.

Strong familial expectations often fuel these myths. In lesbian relationships women must overcome negative messages about their sexual orientation and their sexual practices. Loulan (1984) believes that internalised homophobia can lead to damaged or low self esteem which in turn results in lowered expectations.

Richards' (1990) book along with others highlights a resurgence of interest in identifying positive role models for lesbians. From Sappho and the poetry of the Greek Isles through the salons of Gertrude Stein and Alice Toklas in Paris and Yosano Akiko in Asia to the sculptures of Cath Phillips in Mildura, positive images of lesbians abound. Not only in the arts but also in the sciences are lesbians represented as Richards celebrates 'all their wonderful diversity'. From Agnodice, the first woman gynaecologist in recorded history (4th century BC) to James Miranda Barry, the first English woman doctor (circa 1795) and the Russian mathematician, Sonya Kovalevsky (1850) to the present day pioneers of Phylis Martin and Dell Lyon who founded the first lesbian health centre in San Francisco, lesbians have been prominent in scientific and health care endeavours.

Recently lesbian writers have explored new horizons in female sexuality. Califia (1988) argues that lesbian sex has been viewed too simplistically. Califia believes that socialisation of lesbians has left them frightened to deviate and challenge the status quo in relation to sex and the sexual response:

> Two women in love in a bed who embody all good things the patriarchy is trying to destroy isn't very sexy. This stuff reads as if it were written by dutiful daughters who are trying to persuade Mom that lesbian sex isn't dirty and that we really are good girls, after all.

Menopause

The positive experiences a woman may have in relation to her sexuality may be so tenuous that any change can throw her back into insecurity. The menopausal woman whose body is changing and losing its reproductive function, so integral to status in our society, is particularly at risk. Pfeiffer (1972) found that marital status, age and the enjoyment derived from sex during the younger years influenced women's sexual activity and interest during middle and late years. Hällström's (1979) study of 800 middle aged Swedish women related declining sexual interest in post menopausal women, not to hormonal changes but rather to:

- insufficient emotional support from their partner;
- negative development of relationships;
- poor health of the partner;
- a high number of psychosocial stresses in the past year; and
- unhappiness with work outside the home.

Severne's (1982) study found that socioeconomic class had an influence on menopausal women. High socioeconomic groups reported no emotional or sexual distress, only symptoms related to oestrogen loss whilst lower income women reported the poorest adaptation to all activities of daily life.

Menopausal women may view their changing body and sexual responses as an indication of personal failure. Berkun (1983) reported that menopausal women tend to blame themselves. The medicalisation of the menopause into an endocrine deficiency disorder has on the one hand freed women from victim blaming. Unfortunately it also leaves women wide open to therapeutic and surgical abuse. Hormonal replacement therapy, for example oestrogen and progesterone therapy, whilst alleviating many of the symptoms of menopause, have been linked to breast and uterine cancer. Menstrual irregularities which form a natural part of the ageing process are often treated with invasive techniques such as dilatation and curettage of the uterus and hysterectomy.

Disabled women

Disabled women often find that the Australian culture provides no acknowledgment of their sexual potential. Traditionally they have been discouraged from having sex at all. The social imperative which views disabled mothers as inferior parents is one of the arguments against disabled women engaging in sex. Other arguments include the lack of desire for an 'unattractive' body or the stigma of the spoiled identity as Goffman (1963) calls it and the difficulty in finding suitable physical positions for the sexual act. The tyranny of sexual spontaneity, particularly for women with attendants, also oppresses disabled women.

The sexual responses of disabled women have not been explored. Zwerner (1982), in her studies of sexual issues for women with spinal cord injury, indicates that these women rated sexuality as a high priority and wanted sexual issues included in their total rehabilitation plan. Over half the women in her study had either no change or an increase in their sexual activity after injury. Fitting (1978) in a study of 24 women with spinal cord injuries found that the majority of these women viewed sexual relationships as very enjoyable and very necessary to their adaptation to their acquired disability.

Celibacy

Sexual exploration has led to a greater freedom for women to choose from a variety of possible sexual activities. This freedom of choice has also been accompanied by a freedom to explore a withdrawal from sexual relationships, that is, celibacy. Celibacy may encompass total abstinence from all forms of sexual stimulation, as well as those forms that only relate to the individual woman, e.g. sexual fantasy and masturbation.

Traditionally the reasons for celibacy amongst women have been religious, e.g. the prohibition of premarital sex in some religions and the celibacy of religious orders. More recently, women are finding a period of abstinence as a time for evaluating how important sexual relationships are in their lives. Brown (1980) argues that celibacy 'spiritualises' sexuality, strengthens love relationships and increases physical vitality. Offir (1982) believes that Brown's new celibacy 'sounds suspiciously like old Victorianism'. Finkelstein (1989) believes that sexuality is no longer personal. The meaning of sex has been externalised to conform with societal expectations and not individual needs as she expresses in her memoirs:

I have lost interest in sex. It is like eating Indian or Greek food; I have the aesthetic response but not the bodily. Perhaps it is too much sex over the years, or too little good sex, or too much of other people's sex that has doused my interest. I find myself satiated without having tried it all. It is as if I had secretly gorged myself while in a somnambulistic state or been force-fed by a hungry voyeur. I am no longer moved by penile shaped cars or sofas like women's breasts. I now skim over every mound, cup, curve or rod that is subliminally hidden in my food and clothes.

Without an interest in sex, I began to worry about my mental health, so I took a lover much older thinking that age and experience would bring a new world of sensuality and pleasure. But the urgency of time and the fear of incapacitation made sex a gasping for life. Then, I took a lover much younger, thinking that I could review the ancient process of acquiring sexual tastes, but there were only soft kisses, endless strokes and pats that put me to sleep before waking me up. I have lost interest in sex.

CASE STUDY

She realised she was angry. In fact she was very angry.

She was angry with herself for having been blind to such an issue. She was angry with other women who didn't know, or didn't care enough, or worse still allowed themselves to be exploited. She was angry with men — the power brokers who objectified women, and then derisively dismissed the problem.

What had started out as a whimsical joke a week ago had become a serious issue for Angela.

Angela had always considered herself to be 'together', and aware. After all, at 25, she was a well paid electronics engineer with a multinational company. She was used to working with men, and had been promoted last year ahead of some of her male colleagues. At work, she knew who she was. She was attractive and sensual without being provocative, and two or three of her good male friends at work had told her she was one of the few women they knew who had a very clear view of her own identity — socially, sexually and professionally. Until last week Angela had believed them, and had been rather proud of herself.

Two months ago Angela and Paul decided to get married. They had been living together for two years, and they shared a sense that it was time to move on, to begin thinking about having a family.

They are going to be married in a couple of month's time, and were sitting watching television a week ago, while lazily discussing arrangements for the wedding.

Paul laughed, and kissed Angela, as an ad for soap powder finished. 'Imagine in a year or two, that's what you'll have to become if you're be to a suitable mother for my children.'

'What ARE you talking about?'

'Well, all the ads for things to do with the home have mothers dressed in demure clothes with prim little hairstyles, looking as if they wouldn't know what to do in bed, and couldn't turn on anything except maybe the stove — and of course the shower, to keep their image clean.' Paul smiled at his own joke. He couldn't imagine Angela ever changing or becoming like that. She was far too sensible to be influenced by TV ads anyway.

Angela dismissed the conversation because it was an issue that had never concerned her before. However, later that night her thoughts kept drifting to certain ads, and she began to suspect that Paul might be right.

What was worrying her was that she couldn't understand why she should feel uneasy about all this anyway. What did it matter if marketing techniques used selective images to target their products.

The following night she realised why she was churning over these ideas. She had thought she was very sure of her own sexual identity and her image, but now she seemed to be getting very mixed messages.

On the one hand, the advertising was telling her 'its okay to be sexy, to be provocative and to use your sensuality to your own advantage as long as you are single and sexually uncommitted. As soon as you are committed to one person — especially if you become a wife and mother — you should repress your sexuality, and try to look as asexual as possible.

On the other hand, society's traditional values were saying 'you cannot be sexual until you have an emotional and permanent commitment to one person — especially if you want children. So repress your sexuality until your marriage, and then allow yourself to become instantly sensual and mature, but of course only in the right place at the right time.'

Paul's comments had troubled Angela more than she had wanted to admit at first. Was she really going to change? Was she really as confident of herself and her sexual identity as she thought? How could Paul joke about something so important?

On the train to work the next morning, Angela asked Marg about it. Marg, who worked in the same office block as Angela, had been involved in several feminist organisations — she would straighten things out.

'Where have you been since you left school?', exclaimed Marg, 'Are you for real? Go and buy half a dozen magazines from the newsagent. Buy anything from the Woman's Day to a car magazine and look at the way women are portrayed. There are thousands of subliminal messages about sex out there, all undermining a woman's confidence in her own identity. Do you think they get there by accident? Ads are designed that way, on purpose. People devote a lot of time and skill to giving you and the rest of the world that message. Meet me at lunchtime.'

That began Angela's education. She was amazed that she had never before noticed the model's poses — legs apart, heads back if you were young; legs together, head down or straight ahead, for nonsensual portrayals of professional women, mothers, older women. All the magazines were the same — even those targeting housewives. Other magazines had young girls, twelve and younger in very sensuous poses. Many men's magazines had young women objectified, in very provocative poses trying to sell cars, liquor, computers — the product didn't seem to matter. Angela was stunned at her ignorance and at what was going on.

After that reaction she realised how angry she was. But what could she do about it now ...?

REFERENCES

Ball, M. (1989). *Women and sexuality*, unpublished data.

Berkun, C.S. (1983). *In behalf of women over 40: toward understanding the effect of cessation on women's affective state*, paper presented to Socio-cultural issues in menstrual cycle research, University of California, San Francisco.

Brown, G. (1980). *The new celibacy: why more men and women are abstaining from sex — and enjoying it*, McGraw Hill, New York.

Califa, P., (1988). *Macho sluts*, Alyson Publications, Boston.

Collomb, K. & Howard, M. (1988). Georgia schools help teens postpone sexual involvement, *Georgia medical association journal*, 77(4), 230–232.

de Beauvoir, S. (1972). *The second sex*, Penguin, Harmondsworth.

Ellis, H. (1936). *Prostitution*, vol. IV, Random House, New York.

Finkelstein, J. (1989). Sex in the modern state, in Hawthorne, S. & Pausacker, J., *Moments of desire: sex and sensuality by Australian feminist writers*, Penguin, Victoria.

Finlayson, P., Reynolds, L. & Minn, C. (1987). *Adolescents: their views, problems and needs: a survey of high school students*, Hornsby and Kuring-gai Area Health Services.

Fitting, M.D. (1978). Self concept and sexuality of spinal cord injured women, *Archives of sexual behaviour*, 7, 143–156.

Gagnon, J.H. & Simon, W. (1974). *Sexual conduct: the social sources of human sexuality*, London, Hutchinson.

Goffman, E. (1963). *Stigma: notes on the management of a spoiled identity*, Prentice Hall, New Jersey.

Hällström, T. (1979). Sexuality in women in the middle age: the Goterberg study, *Journal of biosocial science*, supplement, 6, 165–75.

Herschberger, R. (1970). *Adam's rib*, Harper & Row, New York.

Hardy, K. (1964). An appetitional theory of sexual motivation, *Psychological review*, 71, 1–18.

Hite, S. (1976). *The Hite report: a nationwide study of female sexuality*, Dell, New York.

Katchadourian, H.A. (1985). *Fundamentals of human sexuality*, Holt, Rinehart and Winston, New York.

Kinsey, A.C., Pomeroy, W.B. & Martin, C.E. (1948). *Sexual behaviour in the human male*, WB Saunders, Philadelphia.

Kitzinger, S. (1983). *Women's experience of sex*, Penguin, London.

Koutroulis, G. (1990). The orifice revisited: women in gynaecological texts, *Community health studies XIV*, 1, 73–84.

Lockard, D. (1986). The lesbian community: an anthropological approach, *Journal of homosexuality*, 11 (3/4), 83–95.

Loulan, J. (1984). *Lesbian sex*, Spinsters Inc, San Francisco.

McIntosh, M. (1978). Who needs prostitutes? The ideology of male sexual needs, in Smart, C. & Smart, B. *Women, sexuality and social control*, Routledge & Kegan Paul, London.

Mitchell, J. (1974). *Psychoanalysis and feminism*, Allen Lane, London.

National Women's Health Policy (1989). *National women's health policy: advancing women's health in Australia*, AGPS, Canberra.

Offir, C.W. (1982). *Human sexuality*, Harcourt Brace Jovanovich, New York.

Pfeiffer, E., Verwoerdt, A. & Davis, G. (1972). Sexual behaviour in middle life, *American journal of psychology*, 128, 1262–67.

Quadrio, C. (1983). *Anorexia and agoraphobia*, paper presented at the Women in Therapy Conference, ANU, Canberra.

Richards, D. (1990). *Lesbian lists, a look at lesbian culture, history and personalities*, Alyson Publications, Boston.

Richters, J. (1984) Interviews with teenagers, *Healthright*, 3 (3), 22–8.

Severne, L. (1982). Psychosocial aspects of the menopause, in Voda, A., Dinnerstein, M. & O'-Donnell, S. (eds), *Changing perspectives on the menopause*, University of Texas Press, Austin.

Sopchak, A.L. & Sutherland, A.M. (1960). Psychological impact of cancer and its treatment, *Cancer*, 13, 528–531.

The Boston Women's Health Book Collective (1985). *The new our bodies ourselves, a book by women for women*, Penguin, Victoria.

Yerkes, R.M. (1943). *Chimpanzees*, Yale University Press.

Zwerner, J. (1982). Yes we have troubles but nobody's listening: sexual issues of women with spinal cord injury, *Sexuality and disability*, 5, 158–171.

7 Women and Reproduction

Reproductive issues have always been regarded as central to discussions of women's health. The Better Health Commission (1986), for example, was initially limited to considering only those women's health issues which were important in the reproductive years; and of the priorities listed by Newby in the *National women's health policy*, 27 per cent were concerned with reproductive issues. The use of reproduction to describe the way in which women's health needs differ from those of men has frequently been perceived as inappropriate by women as it seems to ignore women's other health needs and to maintain a view of women as mothers, wives and lovers, rather than as people in their own right.

Nonetheless, there are many aspects of women's reproductive life that play a role in determining overall health and well being. It is possible to identify health issues relating to reproduction at each stage of an adult woman's life: in her early reproductive years there may be concerns about menstrual difficulties, contraception and sexually transmitted disease; in her middle reproductive life the issues of childbirth and perhaps infertility may become important; and later there may be concerns about menopause and hysterectomy. This chapter will describe the burden of illness, aetiology and prevention or treatment programs for reproductive issues.

EARLY REPRODUCTIVE LIFE

Menstruation

The onset of menstruation, or menarche, is regarded in many cultures as the beginning of womanhood and may be accompanied by female initiation ceremonies and sometimes betrothal or marriage. In Australia, the average age of menarche is 12.5 years. Over the past century, the onset of menstruation has been occurring at younger ages, probably because of better nutrition and health. Menarche for young women now occurs approximately six months earlier than it did for their mothers, 12 months earlier than it did for their grandmothers and 18 months earlier than it did for their great grandmothers (Bennett 1985). When combined with social changes which have given young women greater freedom and more permission to experiment sexually, the earlier occurrence of menarche has increased the opportunity for adolescent pregnancy.

There are several health issues specifically associated with menstruation, including amenorrhea (lack or cessation of menstruation), dysmenorrhea (painful periods which may be accompanied by nausea), iron-deficiency anaemia, and premenstrual tension or syndrome.

Premenstrual tension has perhaps received the most community interest. The syndrome occurs after the 22nd day of the menstrual cycle, when there are declining levels of sex steroids. The symptoms associated with premenstrual syndrome include bloating, oedema, headache, weight gain, appetite changes, constipation, breast swelling and tenderness, irritability, emotional lability, decreased concentration, anxiety, clumsiness and depression (Russell and Johnson 1987). Problems like schizophrenia and migraine are more likely to occur during the premenstrual phase and rates of asthma, epilepsy, suicide and accidents increase. Precise estimates of the prevalence of premenstrual tension are made difficult by the absence of diagnostic criteria.

Estimates of the prevalence of premenstrual tension vary from 20–40 per cent to 100 per cent of women (Russell and Johnson 1987). A recent study by Redman et al. (1988) found that more than one third of women reported experiencing problems with premenstrual tension and periods during the preceding six months. Abrahams et al. (1985) found that 20 per cent of the young women they surveyed who were aged 14–19 had sought medical advice for menstrual problems.

There are several current theories about the causes of premenstrual tension. These include:

- a progesterone deficiency;
- increased psychoneuroendocrine response to stress;
- decreased catecholamine levels causing depression; and
- changes in prolactin and adrenocortical hormone levels.

There is currently little evidence to indicate which of these theories is more likely to be correct and developing effective treatment strategies is therefore difficult (Russell and Johnson 1987). When treatments have been subjected to adequate evaluation, nutritional and hormonal treatments have been found to be largely ineffective, although there is some evidence that sprionolactone and mefenamic acid (a non-steroidal anti inflammatory agent) can reduce oedema and physical and psychological symptoms respectively (Abrahams and Mira 1986).

Aspects of the health problems associated with menstruation illustrate the relationship between women's health and our health and social institutions. First, as with other aspects of reproductive health, there has been a tendency among health professionals to view health problems associated with menstruation as having a psychogenic cause. Both amenorrhea and dysmenorrhea have been seen as symptoms of women rejecting their womanhood. For example, Lennane and Lennane (1973) quote these descriptions of dysmenorrhea from medical texts

it is generally acknowledged that this condition is much more frequently in the 'high strung', nervous or neurotic female than in her more stable sister.

Faulty outlook ... leading to an exaggeration of minor discomfort ... may even be an excuse to avoid doing something that is disliked.

Second, women are frequently poorly informed about health issues relating to menstruation. Surveys of Australian adolescents indicate that young women poorly understand the changes occurring in their body during menstruation. Sixty one per cent of the young women surveyed by Abrahams et al. (1985) had no idea when in the menstrual cycle ovulation occurred. Further, 75 per cent of the women surveyed considered menstruation to be a 'hassle' and knew little about the correct use of tampons. In the absence of good information, women cannot control their reproductive lives.

Third, in acknowledging that there can be decreases in physical and psychological functioning with different stages in the menstrual cycle, women have felt that they may be laying themselves open to the old criticisms that they are governed by their hormones. In the 'hormonal' view, women are incapable of rational thought premenstrually and behave in an unpredictable manner. Thus women are in a catch 22 situation — if they acknowledge a problem related to menstruation exists they will not be treated as equal to men but if they deny the existence of such problems, they will be unable to seek solutions from the health care system. Fourth, perhaps because of women's ambivalence about drawing attention to menstrual problems and the perception by health care providers that these problems are frequently psychogenic, it is only comparatively recently that much progress has been made in understanding and developing treatment for problems such as dysmenorrhea and premenstrual tension. As a consequence, it seems likely that many women who currently suffer from these problems do not receive adequate treatment, either because they do not ask for help or because the doctor is unaware of treatment options.

It is evident that there is a need to better inform women and health care professionals about health issues relating to menstruation and to better identify women suffering from premenstrual problems. Evaluation of non-pharmacological treatments including counselling and relaxation training is necessary.

Contraception

If women are to control their lives, they need a safe and reliable form of contraception. In the absence of effective and acceptable contraception, it is impossible for women to have the sexual and economic freedoms taken for granted by men or to pursue a life other than that of raising children. To be considered ideal, a contraceptive method needs to:

- provide effective protection from pregnancy;
- have no side-effects, produce no adverse reactions;
- satisfactorily regulate menstruation; and
- be completely acceptable to the user.

Within Australia, four of the most commonly used methods of contraception are the oral contraceptive pill, the IUD, diaphragm, and condom. None of these methods is free from problems.

Khoo (1989) estimates that at least 25 per cent of women of reproductive age in Australia use the Pill. Many women and their doctors believe that the oral contraceptive pill comes closest to fulfilling the requirements of an optimal contraceptive. The Pill has a high success rate (0.1 pregnancies per 100 woman years), does not interrupt love making and appears to be acceptable to users. Early fears that Pill users may have a higher rate of breast cancer appear to be unfounded (Rohan and McMichael 1988), but there does appear to be evidence that the Pill can reduce dysmenorrhoea and irregular menstrual bleeding, and can protect users against benign breast and ovarian cysts in the short term, and endometrial and ovarian cancer in the long term (Khoo 1989).

Nonetheless the Pill does have some important disadvantages. A major problem is the difficulty in remembering to take a pill every day. This is believed to be a particular problem for young women, although studies exploring the characteristics of women who experience Pill failures are rare. The Pill is also unsuitable for women who smoke, those with hypertension, obesity or hyperlipidemia, or those who have suffered a thromboembolism (Khoo 1989). Further, women report a number of side effects of the Pill including reduced libido, mood changes, increased migraine and weight gain (Shearman 1986). However, most empirical studies have not observed a greater prevalence of these problems among women taking the Pill than that observed in the population as a whole (Paul et al. 1986).

Another problem is that a significant number of women still conceive inadvertently while taking the Pill (Khoo 1989). The most common causes of these pregnancies are thought to be missed pills, drug interactions and malabsorption as a result of vomiting or diarrhoea (Kovacs et al. 1989).

Efforts are also presently being made to address some of the short comings of the oral contraceptive pill, by developing various non-oral hormonal contraceptives (Fraser 1988).

Condoms are another commonly used method of contraception. In many ways, condoms represent the ideal contraceptive choice from a women's health perspective. They are easy to use, can be acquired without the need for a doctors appointment, have no side effects, and importantly for women protect against sexually transmitted diseases. The major problem with condoms as a method of contraception is the reluctance of men to use them. Chapman and Hodgson's (1988) study of Australian attitudes towards condom use indicated that many men are opposed to condom use, perceiving condoms as 'pleasure-inhibiting, uncomfortable, unnatural, adolescent, effeminate, unreliable, embarrassing'.

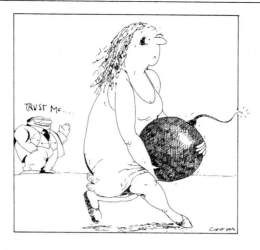

The Dalkon Shield

Some form of contraception is used by most women for much of their reproductive life. The sale of contraception is therefore highly lucrative; women have sometimes felt that a concern with profit from contraception has meant that adequate care to protect their health has not been taken. Claims that drug companies have tested the oral contraceptive pill on third world women and continuing concerns about its long term side effects are examples of a perception that women may be exploited because they need contraception to control their lives. One of the most notorious examples is that of the intrauterine device known as the Dalkon Shield. The following is part of a report by Wendy Bacon published in the *National Times* in 1985:

> A memo sent out by AH Robins' Australian division instructed contraceptive salesmen not to refer to a 1974 United States Food and Drug Administration (FDA) bulletin in their discussions with doctors. The memo was issued by Robins at a time when its Dalkon Shield intrauterine contraceptive device was under investigation in the US. There were about 90 000 women using the shield in Australian at that time.
>
> It has since been accepted that the Dalkon Shield causes a range of complaints including pelvic inflammatory disease, sterility and septic abortion. By 1976, there were 12 deaths in the US directly attributed to it.
>
> Three thousand claims against Robins have resulted in the biggest product liability case in legal history. Robins has already paid out $US233 million in settlements.
>
> The documents relate to the period after June 1974 when AH Robins voluntarily withdrew the Dalkon Shield from the American market. Its decision followed FDA hearings when evidence was given of cases of perforation of the uterine wall, migration of the device into the abdominal wall and the deaths of five pregnant women which were suspected to have been caused by the IUD.
>
> The Australian company failed to withdraw the device from the market at the same time as its parent company. It was not withdrawn here until the following year.
>
> In a later press release justifying the company's decision to keep the IUD on the market the managing director of AH robins in Australia said 'We discussed the matter with Federal health authorities and pointed out that there has been no reported deaths from septic abortion among the 100 000 users in Australia in the four years since it was introduced here.'

Adapted from Wendy Bacon, How Robins shielded the facts on IUD, The *National Times*, February 22–28 1985.

Thus, although condoms have been perceived as offering men an opportunity to be involved in decisions about contraception, Chapman and Hodgson conclude that in the current climate this is unlikely to be an effective method of increasing use rates. They argue that

> whatever reservations one might have about perpetuating the dominant ideology that it should be women's responsibility to attend to contraception ... our material indicates that this is more likely to be a more effective strategy than one that tries to change male reluctance to use condoms.

As a contraceptive method, condoms therefore present a major problem for women — they need to convince their reluctant male partners that they are a good alternative.

Diaphragms are also a useful barrier method of contraception with few side effects. When a diaphragm is used correctly it has a high success rate. Only about 2 per cent of users will have an accidental pregnancy over a year and more than 80 per cent will continue to use the method. However, diaphragms must be inserted before intercourse and left in place for sometime afterwards; they also need to be used with spermicide to be optimally effective. As a result, diaphragms are unacceptable to some women who perceive them as messy, disruptive to lovemaking and removing spontaneity from sexual intercourse.

The fourth commonly used method of contraception is the intrauterine device (IUD). IUDs are acceptable to many women because they avoid the need to consider contraception on a daily basis. Advertised and documented effectiveness rates range from 96–99 per cent. However, controversy over the side effects of intrauterine contraceptive devices has overwhelmed contraceptive debate. These devices function in part by creating inflammation and encouraging infection. Permanent, rather than temporary infertility is often the end result. The technological quest to control the reproduction of the species at any cost is the subject of world wide litigation against the manufacturers of IUDs.

As well as the problems with existing methods of contraception, women frequently do not have enough information about the methods available to make appropriate decisions about contraception. In a study conducted by Children by

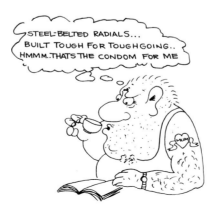

Choice in Queensland (Carmody 1985), for example, one in five teenagers, three quarters of whom were female, reported that they had not heard about condoms, withdrawal or the Pill as methods of contraception. Similarly, it has been estimated in Australia that while 50 per cent of teenage girls are sexually active by the end of high school, only about 10 per cent of these adolescents use any form of birth control. In part, the failure to provide adequate information and skills in contraception to adolescents comes from a belief that young people ought not to be sexually active. This argument comes both from those concerned with the morality of sexual intercourse outside of marriage and those who believe that teenagers are too young and too vulnerable to engage in sexual intercourse.

Priorities for women's health in the area of contraception therefore include the development of more effective methods of contraception and the provision of adequate information about contraception to all women capable of conceiving.

Unwanted pregnancy

Failure to provide adequate information about contraception will result in unwanted pregnancies. The Royal Commission on Human Relationships, 1977 estimated that 15 per cent of nuptial births and 30 per cent of exnuptial births in Australia are unwanted. There is some evidence of long term negative consequences for a child of being unwanted, including an increased likelihood of social and psychological problems in later life (Pohlman 1969). It has been estimated that 85 per cent of marriages occurring because the woman is pregnant break up within five years (Holmes 1985) and women who are single parents are one of the poorest groups in Australian society.

A high proportion of unwanted pregnancies occur among teenage women. Although teenage fertility rates have decreased in the past decade, at least 5 per cent of women aged between 15 and 19 became pregnant in 1982 — a total of 33 196 teenage pregnancies (Holmes 1985). Holmes estimates that between 10 and 15 per cent of total births occur to teenage mothers, some as young as 12 years of age. The consequences of adolescent pregnancy can be great for both mother and child. There may be physical risks to the mother because of the immaturity of her body and also to the child (Stanley and Straton 1981). Social risks include failure to complete schooling or job training and likely poverty (Furstenburg et al. 1989).

Although the lack of an effective method of contraception contributes to unwanted pregnancy, the absence of good information about and easy access to contraception among adolescents is likely to be more important. Jones (1985) undertook a cross cultural comparison of teenage pregnancy rates. She showed that the pregnancy rate in Sweden was 20 per 1000 women compared with rates of 62 in the USA and 27 in England and Wales. She argued that a higher rate of teenage pregnancy occurred in countries in which there was a high degree of reported religiosity, poor availability of contraceptive education in schools, poor access to counselling, and education programs directed at morality rather than those designed to prevent pregnancy.

Abortion

For those women who have an unwanted pregnancy, there are only two options — to continue with the pregnancy or to have an abortion. Abortion has historically been the most common form of birth control, and it has been estimated that one in four pregnancies are aborted on a global basis (Holmes 1985). When abortions are undertaken in appropriate clinics, or by skilled professionals, and before the end of the first six weeks of pregnancy, the health risks to the woman are very low. Further, a number of studies appear to indicate that for the majority of women abortion poses no threat to their mental or physical well being. Relief appears to be the most predominant initial emotion and few women report grief or depression over the next few months (Holmes 1985).

There are perhaps few women's health issues that have caused as much debate as abortion. Advocates of abortion have argued that women have a right to control their bodies and therefore that abortion should be readily available to women who find themselves pregnant when they do not wish to be so. The main issues are perceived to be those of availability and safety. In contrast, opponents of abortion argue that human life begins at conception and that women do not therefore have the right to decide to end another human beings life (Coombs 1985).

In practice, the second view has more frequently been dominant. The abortion laws in Australia are derived from the English laws which made abortion illegal. These laws offered relatively mild penalties, regarding abortion before quickening as about as serious a crime as buggery, and equating abortion after quickening with arson of farm buildings (Hurse 1985). Because of the poor sanitary conditions under which abortions were undertaken, there was a high rate of complications and many women died. In understanding the legal position, it is important to note that abortion laws were initially introduced to protect the woman rather than the fetus. Although all states in Australia have laws against abortion, the laws and their implementation differ from state to state. The differences hinge on the conditions under which abortion is legal and the interpretation of these clauses. In Queensland for example, abortion was made illegal in 1899, although a legal loophole was provided by the clause which allowed abortions to preserve the mother's life. This clause was intended to permit doctors to save the mother's life during a difficult birth but has been used in Victoria and NSW to allow women access to abortion on a wide range of grounds. Elsewhere in Australia the clause has not been tested. Currently, in NSW and Victoria, abortion is legal to preserve the mother's physical or mental health on reasonable grounds which may be economic, social or medical and so, in practice, abortion is available upon request. In other states, Queensland in particular, abortion is much more difficult to obtain and the interpretation of the law less clear.

Sexually transmitted diseases (STDs)

Sexually transmitted diseases (STDs) are also of importance to women in their early reproductive years, since they are major causes of infertility and other health problems (Clark 1985; NH & MRC working party report 1988b). Many STDs are symptomless in women and therefore are not detected early enough to prevent damage. Although many STDs are notifiable, the surveillance system is currently inadequate and therefore it is difficult to estimate even the prevalence of many STDs among women. The NH & MRC Working Party on pelvic inflammatory disease (PID), for example, believed that under-reporting was a significant problem. They estimate that under-reporting may be of the order of 90 per cent for gonorrhoea and higher for non-specific utheritis. Studies in the Northern Territory and in Queensland (Douglas, Greenoff and Woodroffe 1984–6; Smithurst and Armstrong 1975; Sexually transmitted disease surveillance 1982) have found that sexually transmitted diseases are most common in women under 25 and women in lower socioeconomic groups. Aboriginal women were also found to have a high incidence of chlamydial infection.

Discussion of STDs in relation to women's health has focussed particularly on the risk posed by chlamydia and associated PID, and AIDs.

Chlamydia is a health problem for women because of the association between this disease and subsequent infertility. Chlamydia is usually symptomless but may be associated with vaginal discharge, dysuria, pelvic pain and in neonates, conjunctivitis and pneumonia. Among a sample of women attending the Royal Women's Hospital, 83 per cent of those with infertility due to inflammatory tubal disease or ectopic pregnancy had had chlamydia infections, most of them repeated infections (Garland and Johnson 1989). Only 10 per cent of pregnant women and 7 per cent of women with infertility due to other causes had had chlamydia infections. A recent examination of a sample of 1000 women attending a Family Planning Association Clinic outside Sydney found chlamydia to be present in 5.1 per cent of the women (Kovacs et al. 1988), and studies at other family planning clinics suggest that between 5 and 10 per cent of women have unsuspected chlamydia infections.

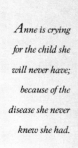

Anne is crying for the child she will never have; because of the disease she never knew she had.

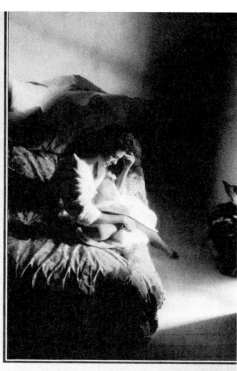

An advertisement aimed at general practitioners, promoting improved detection and treatment of chlamydia

Chlamydia can be detected using a simple test and treatment in the early stages is highly effective (Gilbert 1987). There are currently a number of moves at the public health level to improve the situation for women in terms of chlamydia. There are calls to make it a notifiable disease which, even given current levels of underreporting, would highlight the importance of chlamydia infections. There are currently major education campaigns targeted at general practitioners underway to improve their awareness of the prevalence and potential consequences of chlamydia infections.

Consequences of the Acquired Immune Deficiency Syndrome (AIDS) for women must also be considered. Although AIDS is still relatively uncommon among women, accounting for only 3.2 per cent of cases diagnosed in Australia up until September 1989, the prevalence is expected to increase. Many women remain at risk of infection through their use of intravenous drugs, by having unprotected intercourse with men who use intravenous drugs, and/or with bisexual men (Philpot et al. 1988). Prevention for women involves similar measures as for men namely avoiding sharing needles and using condoms during intercourse.

MIDDLE REPRODUCTIVE LIFE

During the middle period of a woman's reproductive life, issues include those associated with pregnancy and childbirth, for some women infertility will be a problem and it is important that women establish regular patterns of screening for cervical cancer.

Pregnancy and childbirth

Perhaps not surprisingly, much more is known about pregnancy and childbirth than any of the other reproductive issues described in this chapter. During the 18th and 19th centuries, pregnancy was regarded as a healthy and normal state. On average, a peasant woman gave birth within a year after marriage and every two years thereafter until menopause (Branca 1978). She therefore spent at least 15 years of her life bearing children and recovering from childbirth. Women were attended during childbirth by midwives. Midwifery skills were acquired by experience and informal apprenticeship. Some midwives received extensive training (Mitchell and Oakley 1976). However, by the end of the 19th century, male doctors were taking an increasing interest in pregnancy and childbirth (see chapter one). The move from predominantly midwife care to predominantly doctor care was rapid, particularly among the middle classes. In Great Britain, by 1946 less than 15 per cent of women received their antenatal care from midwives compared with 100 per cent at the turn of the century (Enkin and Chalmers 1982). The move was fostered by an increased interest in science and scientific approaches among the middle classes and represented a move from a community of apparently untrained or informally trained women to a profession of formally trained men. Along with the move from midwife to obstetrician, there was an increasing emphasis on antenatal care: in Great Britain, the number of pregnant women who received antenatal care at the turn of the century was negligible, but by 1935 it was estimated that 80 per cent of expectant mothers received antenatal care of some kind almost half of them in state aided clinics.

Figure 7.1: Maternal mortality in Australia and the United Kingdom

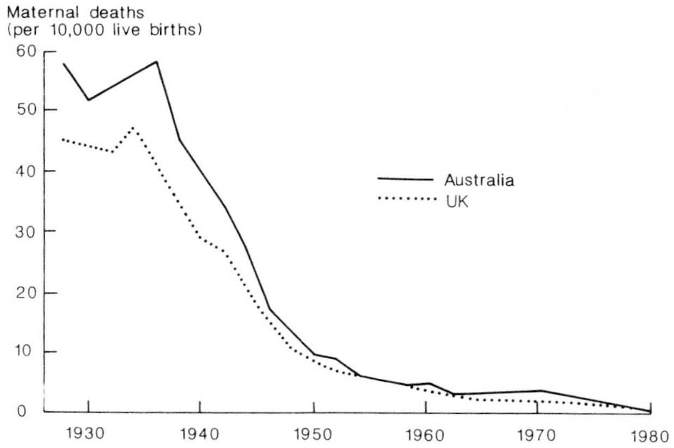

(Llewellyn-Jones 1986)

A little later childbirth became further medicalised with the trend towards increasing provision of maternity care in hospitals, rather than in community settings. All women are now encouraged to deliver their babies in hospital (Enkin and Chalmers 1982). Thus, pregnancy has increasingly become an 'illness' requiring highly specialised treatment and supervision within a medical setting.

During this period there was however a dramatic fall in maternal and infant mortality as shown in figure 7.1. Childbirth is no longer a major cause of death for women and the fall in infant mortality has meant that most women have fewer pregnancies. The reasons for the fall in maternal and infant mortality are complex. Initially the greater use of technology and specialist care was seen as primarily responsible (Illich 1976). However, it now seems likely that improvements in nutrition, education and public health have done as much to lower the death rate during pregnancy and child birth as improved obstetric technology.

The historical development of care provided during pregnancy and childbirth has left us today with a series of problems. First, it is increasingly argued that the medicalisation of childbirth has led to too great a rate of intervention during childbirth. Many people believe that childbirth ought to occur naturally for most women and that existing rates of interventions such as induction, forceps delivery and caesarian section are too high. Modern hospital obstetric practices include invasive diagnostic procedures, induction and acceleration of labour, reliance on drugs for pain relief, routine electrical foetal monitoring, high caesarian section rates, and separation of the mother and baby after birth. British figures demonstrate the increasing level of intervention, showing that the average number of antenatal tests and procedures being carried out rose from around three per cent in the 1950s, to ten per cent in the 1970s, while the percentage of inductions also rose dramatically over the same period from 8 per cent to 24 per cent (Enkin and Chalmers 1982). Australian figures demonstrate a large geographical variation in intervention which strongly suggest that many interventions during labour and delivery are determined by the attendant obstetrician rather than the needs of the

mother (Maternity Services in NSW 1989). The high levels of intervention in pregnancy and childbirth have been the focus of complaints about the medicalisation
of women's reproductive health, and a rejection to some degree, of the medical
model which treats birth as an illness (Lewin and Olesen 1985). The widespread
use of a number of the common modern obstetric practices, such as the induction
and acceleration of labour are now considered to be of questionable value (Holmes, Hoskings and Gross 1980).

Second, there has been increasing evidence that many women are dissatisfied
with maternity services. Many women believe that maternity care does not provide
them with sufficient opportunity to control what happens to them and that the
staff do not provide enough information about what is happening. The recent
report of the Ministerial Task Force on Obstetric Services in NSW emphasised the
need for maternity care services to be more flexible and promote each woman's
informed participation in decisions during pregnancy and childbirth. Expanding
the role of the midwife and the use of birth centres were identified by the task force
as ways of providing more balanced and acceptable antenatal and maternity care.
It has been found that in birth centres, the intervention rates are lower, and the
outcomes for both mother and baby are as good or better than are those for

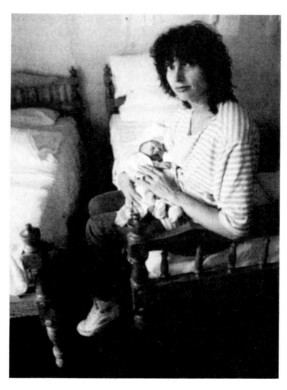

Birthing centre at the Royal Women's Hospital, Paddington

women of comparative risk in a labour ward (Bennett and Shearman 1989). It may also be that attendance at antenatal education classes can help increase satisfaction with childbirth by increasing the women's knowledge of what is likely to happen and the choices available to her. Antenatal classes can also help involve the father in childbirth.

Third, it has been argued that the concern with maternal and infant mortality has persisted long after these have been major issues for women. Currently, within Australia, maternal mortality rates associated with childbirth are no longer a major cause for concern, as deaths due to direct obstetric causes have shown a significant decrease to the current level of 0.13 per 1000 confinements (NH & MRC 1988a). Morbidity of some kind is however, experienced by most if not all women during pregnancy and childbirth (Harrison 1985) and warrants greater concern from health care providers. Backache for example is experienced by 48 per cent of women, while soft tissue trauma, ranging from minimal to gross bruising and swelling to lacerations and/or episiotomy is common during childbirth, as is muscle weakness and fatigue and tension. Ten to fifteen per cent of women are also found to experience post-natal depression which may last for several months and impair a woman's ability to function (O'Hara 1987; O'Hara, Neuraber and Zekoski 1984).

Increased attention to preventive health issues may also increase maternal and infant well being. For example, Harrison (1985) cites evidence that correct advice and training given in antenatal and postnatal preparation and education classes significantly reduces some forms of maternal morbidity, such as severe backache, muscle weakness, and fatigue and tension. Encouraging women to stop smoking during pregnancy and to continue breast feeding their babies will decrease infant morbidity.

Infertility

The causes of infertility are varied, and are estimated to affect 10 to 15 per cent of heterosexual couples (Brown 1985). Approximately one third of infertility relates to health problems in the woman, one-third to problems in the man and the remainder to a combination of problems between the two (Brown 1985).

Brown reports that the major causes of infertility in women are endometriosis and tubal blockages. Other known causes included undiagnosed and untreated appendicitis in young women, contraception (especially IUD's which can cause pelvic inflammatory diseases), and sexually transmitted diseases.

The in vitro fertilisation (IVF) procedure is currently the most successful strategy for dealing with infertility. IVF however, is suitable to redress only about 25 per cent of all cases of infertility and incurs a high financial and emotional cost (Australian in-vitro fertilization collaborative group 1988; Best 1988). The process also has a high failure rate. The chances of a live birth in each treatment cycle were below 10 per cent and only 57.5 per cent of those treatments resulting in a pregnancy proceeded to a live birth. Therefore, it seems that the most cost-effective way of dealing with infertility is to attempt to detect and prevent sexually transmitted diseases, and to develop reliable forms of contraception which do not have detrimental effects on a woman's fertility.

There also appears to be a need for much improved support services for those who go through the IVF programme, whether the intervention is successful or not

IVF: a one-woman issue

'The doctors were pigs. They showed no compassion. It was an emotionally destroying experience.'

This was how a friend described her time on an IVF program in England. At the end of several tries, she abandoned the program — without a baby — among the overwhelming majority for whom the technology fails.

Superficially, she sounds like the contributors to a new book edited by Renate Klein, of Deakin University, Geelong, called *Infertility: Women speak out about their experiences of reproductive medicine* (Pandora).

In the book, women from many countries describe what they endure when the pursuit of motherhood takes over their lives. For a long time they will put up with any amount of pain and debasement to try to have a child of their own. Their marriages, their work, their studies grind to a halt as they try one 'fix' after another.

Increasingly, feminists have spoken out against IVF, characterising it as a technology which exploits women and rarely gives them what they want — a baby.

Unfortunately the critics have come to sound condescending and authoritarian, no better, often, than the anti-abortion brigade which also seeks to limit women's choices. In calling for international resistance to IVF, feminists critics are really saying 'we want to protect women from themselves. We know the technology is dangerous and dehumanising but other women, the ones who queue up to try, have somehow failed to realise it.'

My friend who underwent IVF knows all about the stress, the constant uncertainty, the fear of long-term side effects from the hormones, the time-tabled sex and the emptiness at the end, but still says, 'I don't regret it. I would tell another woman what it was like for me and then I would say, go ahead, try it, you might be one of the lucky ones.'

The critics ignore women like her. They assume women rush into IVF in a thoughtless manner, ignorant of the pain, disruption and intervention entailed, and blind to the program's failure rate.

They often ascribe women's overwhelming need to have their own children to social pressures. In short, they see the women as needing to be saved from their own despair, ignorance and cultural conditioning. This notion of the helpless female does not apply to the two women I know, who are soon to embark, eyes open, on IVF.

As much as anyone can be prepared for pain and failure, they are prepared. Of course the preparation may not save them from despair; no more than the well-informed pregnant woman may be guaranteed an easy labour.

But they have already tasted so much pain and heartache that another blow, they believe, will not finish them off. 'I can't feel much worse than I do,' one said.

She has decided to embark on IVF after two years of self-searching during which she has asked profound and difficult questions.

As for IVF's medical horrors, my friend believes her experience to date — incompetent doctors, mis-diagnosis, two ectopic pregnancies — are ample preparation. Like many on IVF after similar experiences, she is under no illusion about medical science or manners. Yet she still wants to proceed.

Both the women who have opted for IVF are feminist, well-travelled career women. Cultural conditioning does not entirely explain their fierce desires to have children. They know a woman does not have to be a mother to be worthwhile, but still they want to be mothers.

Another woman I know went to an IVF counselling session and was so appalled that she immediately decided it was not for her. It was her decision. Surely this is how it should be. Women are not fools.

And society pays one way or another through subsidising psychiatrists' bills or through subsidising the technology.

The IVF critics may help bring about better counselling, more information and better doctors. Their total opposition, however, risks fabricating two classes of infertile women — the worthies who 'resist' IVF and to whom Klein dedicates her book — and the rest, by implication, weak and foolish.

Perhaps my friend is wrong and she may feel much, much worse, but who are we to say her pain is not worth the try?

Adele Horin, *Sydney Morning Herald*, 8 August 1989.

(Brown 1985). Brown also suggests that there is perhaps an even greater need to help infertile women to accept and cope with their condition, rather than putting them through the expensive, traumatic and largely unsuccessful IVF procedure. Research is required to establish the best ways of providing support and assistance to both these groups of women.

Figure 7.2: Percentage of women attending general practitioners having a Pap smear in the last 3 years

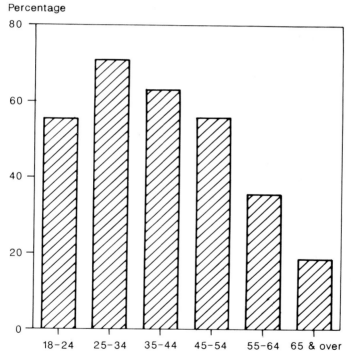

(Based on Dickinson et al. 1988)

Cervical cancer

Each year according to the Australasian Association of Cancer Registries (1987), 350 women die from cervical cancer and almost 1000 cases of invasive disease are diagnosed in Australia. The incidence of cervical cancer increases with age and reaches a peak among women aged 55–64 (Office of Population Censuses Surveys 1983); there is also a link between sexual behaviour and cervical cancer as women who have never been sexually active do not develop the disease and risk increases with number of sexual partners (Hulka 1982).

Cervical cancer is almost entirely preventable by routine Papanicolaou (Pap) smears. These smears detect premalignant abnormalities in the cervix which can be treated to prevent the development of cervical cancer. Overseas studies have shown that both the incidence and mortality from cervical cancer can be reduced by screening programs (Hakama et al. 1985).

Within Australia, there is currently no national cervical cancer screening program. Most smears are provided by general practitioners although women's health nurses, gynaecologists and family planning organisations also provide smears. There is a considerable debate about the appropriate frequency of screening for cervical cancer within Australia. In 1988, the Australian Cancer Council recommended the following for cervical screening (Fleming 1985):

- all women should be screened;
- screening should commence at 18;
- screening should stop at 65 provided that all previous smears have been normal;
- after two normal annual smears, three year screening is recommended.

However, more recently the Royal College of General Practitioners have recommended annual screening for all women.

Despite the advantages of screening for cervical cancer, many Australian women are currently not appropriately screened. Estimates of the proportion of women adequately screened vary depending on the population and data source used. Mitchell and Medley (1987), for example, reported that 18 per cent of women were receiving an annual smear based on estimates from pathology records, while Bowman et al. (1990a) found that 75 per cent reported that they had had a smear in the previous three years. Of particular concern is the consistent finding that older women who are most at risk of developing cervical cancer have the poorest rates of Pap smears. Mitchell and Medley, for example, report that while 26 per cent of women in the 30–39 year age group had had a smear in the previous year, only 13 per cent of women aged 50–59 and 7 per cent of women aged between 60 and 65 had had a smear. Other studies have reported similar findings (see figure 7.2).

Several factors may be important in explaining why many women do not currently receive regular Pap smears. Surveys of women and doctors have highlighted the central importance of general practitioners in ensuring that regular screening occurs. For example, in a survey of New Zealand women the most frequent reason given for having had a recent smear was that the doctor had recommended it (Bailie and Petrie 1990). However, it is evident that since most women attend their doctor within a one year period, general practitioners currently miss many opportunities to offer Pap smears to women. One reason for this may be a lack of clear recommendations about Pap smears. In a recent survey of general practitioners, Bowman et al. (1990b) found that many were confused about who was eligible for Pap smears with 50 per cent believing inappropriately that Pap smears were necessary for women who had never had intercourse and for women who had had a hysterectomy. Perhaps not surprisingly given the

The unfortunate experiment

Women's lack of control over their reproductive lives is evident in many of the topics discussed in this chapter. Some of the critical issues are illustrated by the events surrounding a research program into cervical cancer carried out at the National Women's Hospital in Auckland, New Zealand. Usually, when women present with premalignant abnormalities of the cervix such as carcinoma in situ, the lesions are removed to prevent them developing into invasive cancer. However, during the 1970s women attending the National Women's Hospital with carcinoma in situ were part of a study into the natural history of cervical cancer; the doctors believed that carcinoma in situ did not develop into invasive cancer and some of the women were therefore given no treatment for their condition. All women were given a Pap smear test at the end of diagnosis, whether or not they had been treated. Follow up of the women who were part of this study indicated that whether or not they had been treated, 1.5 per cent of the women who had negative smears after diagnosis developed invasive cancer, while 22 per cent of the women who had positive smears developed invasive cancer. Coney comments that the rate of cervical cancer among those women with positive smear tests was 25 times that of the women with negative tests. The development of cervical cancer was particularly high among those women who were offered no treatment and returned positive smears with 90 per cent developing invasive cancer.

The conduct of this study raises a number of issues. First, the failure to treat women with cancer in situ was contrary to treatment practices elsewhere in the world at the time. In Australia and other hospitals in New Zealand the results of large scale evaluative studies were accepted as showing that the treatment of premalignant abnormalities in the cervix would decrease the rate of development of invasive cancer. The women who were part of the National Women's Hospital study were therefore denied treatment that would normally have been provided and as a result of the absence of treatment many of them died from invasive cervical cancer. Second, the women were unaware that they were part of a clinical trial; most of the women appeared to believe that they were being provided with optimal care and that the absence of treatment meant that they were not in danger of developing cancer. At no point did the women consent to being part of a research study and it is doubtful that many would have given their consent if they were aware of the potential consequences of not receiving treatment. Third, the follow up procedures were less than optimal. It is clear that there was sufficient information about the consequences of no treatment to end the trial a long time before it did finish. In fact, the no-treatment arm of the trial became routine hospital practice without a thorough examination of the outcome for the women enrolled in the study. Moreover, even when the results of the trial became known, the hospital made little attempt to follow up the women who had been in the no–treatment arm and had untreated carcinoma in situ.

As part of the subsequent inquiry into this research project, it became evident that the importance of informed consent was not at all well understood by the participating doctors. The inquiry also revealed that at the same hospital, anaesthetised women were frequently used to teach medical students how to perform vaginal vault examinations — obviously without their consent! Further, Pap smears were taken from a large number of newborn baby girls without their parents consent. These Pap smears were again used for research purposes; they were used to assess whether premalignant cervical abnormalities are present from birth.

Adapted from, S. Coney, *The unfortunate experiment*, Penguin Books, 1988.

conflicting recommendations about Pap smears, many of the general practitioners surveyed were also confused about the most appropriate screening frequency. Another reason for the low rates of screening may be a reluctance on the part of women to have Pap smears; the general practitioners in Bowman et al.'s study believed that the rates of Pap smear screening could be increased if women were better informed and more assertive about requesting smears. The embarrassment of the test was cited frequently in Bailie and Petrie's survey as a reason for women not initiating Pap smears. A further cause of the low screening rates may be that it is difficult for both general practitioners and women to remember about the need for regular Pap smears. In the Bailie and Petrie study the most frequently reported reason that women gave for not having a Pap smear test was that they had not got around to having the test. Centralised reminder systems such as that operated by the New South Wales Cancer Council may therefore do much to increase screening rates.

Encouraging both women and their doctors to ensure that Pap smears are undertaken on a regular basis is a major challenge in women's health since it has the potential to save the lives of many women.

LATE REPRODUCTIVE LIFE

Older women have claimed that once they are no longer capable of bearing children, there is little interest in their reproductive problems among either doctors or the community in general. It is increasingly recognised that the problems relating to reproductive issues in later life are critical in ensuring the overall health and quality of life of women. The issues of menopause and hysterectomy have received particular attention.

Menopause

About 20 per cent of menopausal women have some physical symptoms severe enough for them to seek medical attention, according to the *Report of the public health service task force on women's health issues* (1985). Menopause has a number of major detrimental effects on women's health, including causing osteoporosis, vaginal irritation and dysuria due to atrophy of urogenital tissues and vasomotor rushes (hot flushes). Psychological changes such as a greater incidence of depression, fatigue, irritability and negative moods have also been noted (Armstrong 1988; WHO Scientific Group 1981).

Osteopororis is seen to be one of the most important concomitants of menopause, affecting approximately 25 per cent to 30 per cent of all post menopausal women (Angus and Eisman 1988). In addition to causing deformity and discomfort through its effects on the spine, osteoporosis is a major cause of fracture of the long bones. It is estimated that one in five women in Australia will suffer a fracture related to osteoporosis by the age of 75 (Sambrook and Eisman 1989).

The medical management of the problems associated with menopause has centred on the use of oestrogen replacement therapy and calcium supplements for osteoporosis. Oestrogen therapy has demonstrated beneficial effects for postmenopausal women. However, its use carries risks, such as increased likelihood of developing endometrial cancer and cardiovascular disease. Further, osteoporosis cannot be completely effectively treated with hormone replacement and calcium supplements. Prevention, through the use of health education programs encouraging correct nutrition and regular weight-bearing exercise, appears to be the only really effective way of combating osteoporosis.

Hysterectomy

Approximately 19 per cent of Australian women in the 40–64 age group have undergone a hysterectomy. Hysterectomies are provided for cancers of the womb or genital tract, fibroids, prolapse and bleeding and pain. Most women who have hysterectomies report improved quality of life as a result of the absence of pain and bleeding. However, hysterectomy is a major operation which carries a risk of death (Dicker et al. 1982). There is also the risk of secondary complication following hysterectomy; the rates of secondary complications are estimated to be between 25 per cent and 50 per cent (Easterday, Grimes and Riggs 1983). Complications of the procedure include: secondary haemorrhage, severe or recurring urinary tract infection, incisional hernia, sepsis, intestinal obstruction, poor appetite and constipation (Sandberg et al. 1985). Psychiatric problems such as depression may also occur, although recent prospective studies suggest that psychological morbidity may be less than previously suggested (Sandberg et al. 1985).

Hysterectomy rates have been found to vary across time, geographic region and by age and socioeconomic status of the patient (Illich 1976). Perhaps of most interest is the geographic variations: the hysterectomy rate in the USA and Canada for example is three times the rate in Britain with Australian rates falling midway between the two (Schacht and Pemberton 1985). Studies have also shown a wide variation in hysterectomy rates in different areas in Australia. Daniel (1985), for example, reported that the rates of hysterectomy standardised for age and compared with a rate across New South Wales of 100, was 132 in the Hunter Region compared with 77 in New England. Up to 90 per cent of hysterectomies are elective, and variations in rate cannot be accounted for by variations in the incidence and risk of uterine disease. Therefore, there is concern that in regions where the rate is high, women may be encouraged to have a hysterectomy when it may not be essential. Differences between the rebates offered to doctors within different systems have been thought to partly account for the international variations in hysterectomy rates among countries which are similar in terms of the health status of their populations. Since the rebate to the gynaecologist is good, it has been argued that doctors need hysterectomies more than their women patients.

It is therefore necessary to better inform patients of the possible risks, costs and benefits associated with having a hysterectomy. Providing a stronger basis on which women might make the decision whether or not to have a hysterectomy, may also help to decrease psychological morbidity following the procedure (Neefus and Taylor 1981).

ISSUES IN REPRODUCTION

There have been some particular problems in ensuring that women receive adequate and acceptable health care in relation to reproductive issues. First, there has

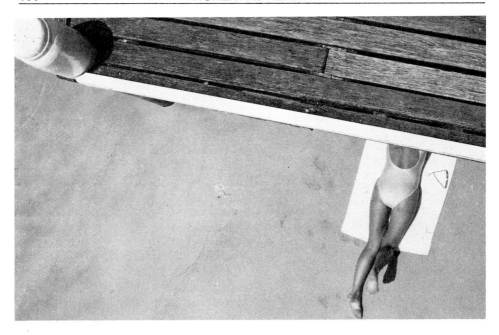

The picture above advertises a popular brand of contraceptive pill. Compare this image with that portrayed in the picture below, an advertisement for hormone replacement therapy. No longer young and 'available', menopause is a period of grief and a premonition of death.

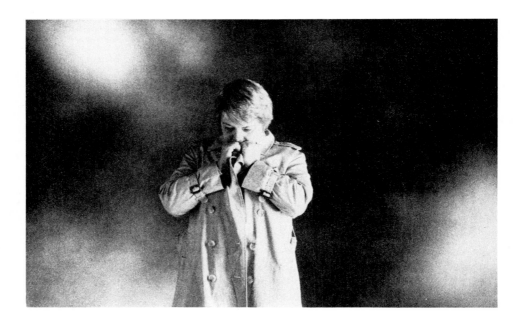

frequently been a tension between the perception that reproductive issues are the normal functions of a healthy woman and the view that the reproductive process should involve doctors or other health care workers. The process of involving health care workers has been seen as the medicalisation of healthy women, but has been the dominant philosophy throughout much of this century. It is illustrated by the move from midwife to obstetrician care during pregnancy and labour, the replacement of 'natural' methods of contraception such as withdrawal and the rhythm method by medical management based on the contraceptive pill or intrauterine devices and the high rates of hysterectomy. In the last fifteen years, the women's health movement has expressed increasing opposition to the medicalisation of reproductive issues.

Second, it is evident that women have frequently lacked control of their reproductive health. Women have been provided with insufficient information about contraception to control their fertility and prevented from obtaining safe abortions when they believed that this was the most appropriate choice for them. Although the move from midwife care and home deliveries to obstetrician care and hospital deliveries contributed to the decrease in infant and maternal mortality, it represented a loss of control over childbirth for many women. The failure to obtain consent for the National Women's Hospital study of cervical cancer is another example of our failure to allow women to control their reproductive health.

Third, there is a perception that many reproductive issues of importance to women have not been given sufficient priority within the health care system. In particular, it has been argued that issues such as premenstrual tension, changes during menopause and problems such as pelvic inflammatory disease have been largely ignored by the health care system, and insufficient care has been provided for problems which require routine screening or counselling. The health care system has been seen as slow to react to the changing focus of women's reproductive health needs. The decline of maternal and child mortality during childbirth has shifted the focus in this area to issues of quality of life and morbidity. With the exception of cervical cancer, the majority of women's health issues currently relate to reducing morbidity rates rather than increasing life expectancy. The health care system therefore needs to supply programs for detecting these problems and appropriate management strategies.

CASE STUDY

All night Anna was restless. It was hot and she couldn't get back to sleep. At four o'clock in the morning she felt her first real contraction. While it was uncomfortable, it was also very exciting. She woke Brian, who got up and began to think through the months and months of preparation for the next few hours. Anna had practised relaxation and they had prepared tapes of music. They had planned a home birth and set up the living room with specially arranged lighting.

Two or three hours later the midwife Helen arrived. Anna was having regular contractions, some of them quite painful. But Helen said there was quite a long time to go because her cervix had not dilated beyond two centimetres. The cervix would need to be dilated to ten centimetres for the baby's head to pass through.

By lunchtime, Brian was not very happy. Anna was in a lot of pain and though she was coping well, it was hard to watch her suffering and every contraction seemed so long. He didn't like the way Helen was hovering around. She was obviously anxious.

Because they had had lots of conversations in the past, he felt he knew her well enough to ask 'What's up Helen? Is this what it's supposed to be like?' Helen always believed in clear communication with patients, but had been hesitating because she knew how much Anna and Brian wanted a home birth. She told them that Anna's labour was not progressing as it should and that she would advise them to go to hospital now. She would still be able to continue supervising the delivery, but a monitor would check the baby's progress.

In spite of her increasing pain and frustration, Anna was very disappointed and very reluctant to leave home. She accused Helen of not being competent to deal with a small complication. Patiently Helen emphasised the baby's need for oxygen and the complexity of the birthing process. While she acknowledged Anna's intense disappointment and fear about going to hospital, she stated clearly that her professional advice was to seek immediate obstetric care.

Half an hour later they were in the labour ward of their local hospital. Brian made sure they had some music and a camera to photograph the birth. The nurses were kind but seemed a bit put out that the hospital was only seen as second best and were impatient with Anna's request to have music on. An hour later the monitor that had been placed on the baby showed that it was experiencing distress, that is a lack of oxygen, and Anna's cervix was still not fully dilated.

Then everything happened at once. An obstetrician, whom neither Anna nor Brian had met, came in and, after a brief discussion and examination, agreed to do a Caesarean section. He was rather off-hand and clearly not pleased to be involved only at the last minute. It was difficult to find an anaesthetist, as two other emergency operations were in progress at the same time. In the middle of all this Anna whispered to Brian 'What are they doing? They seem to have forgotten that this is our baby and our experience. Don't they realise we've been planning this for months?'

Before Brian could even answer, he was whisked out the door by the Sister and told firmly he could not attend the Caesarean operation. Impatient and angry, he paced the waiting room outside.

Moments later a young nurse came out smiling and asked him, 'Can you hear that baby crying? That's your daughter.'

All kinds of feelings began to overwhelm him......

REFERENCES

Abraham, S. & Mira, M. (1986). Premenstrual syndrome: new strategies for treatment, *Current therapeutics*, 27 (8), 51–61.

Abraham, S., Fraser, I., Gebski, V., Knight, C., Llewellyn-Jones, D., Mira, M. & McNeil, D. (1985). Menstruation, menstrual protection and menstrual cycle problems, *The medical journal of Australia*, 142, 247–251.

Angus, R.M. & Eisman, J.A. (1988). Osteoporosis: the role of calcium intake and supplementation, *The medical journal of Australia*, 149, 630–633.

Armstrong, B.K. (1988). Oestrogen therapy after the menopause — boon or bane? *The medical journal of Australia*, 148, 213–214.

Australasian Association of Cancer Registries & Australian Institute of Health (1987). Cancer in Australia, in Giles, G.G., Armstrong, B.K. & Smith, L.R. (eds) *National cancer statistics*, Clearing House Publication No. 1.

Australian in-vitro fertilization collaborative group, (1988). IVF pregnancies in Australia and New Zealand, *The medical journal of Australia*, 148, 429–436.

Bailie, R. & Petrie, K. (1990). Women's attitudes to cervical smear testing, *New Zealand medical journal*, 103, 293–5.

Bennett, D.L. (1985). Menarche — a major milestone to womanhood, *The medical journal of Australia*, 142, 244–245.

Bennet, C. & Shearman, R. (1989). Maternity services in NSW — childbirth moves toward the 21st century, *The medical journal of Australia*, 150, 673–676.

Best, J. (1988). Avoiding throwing the baby out with the bath water, *The medical journal of Australia*, 149, 97–102.

Better Health Commission (1986). *Looking forward to better health*, vol. 3, AGPS, Canberra.

Bowman, J., Redman, S., Dickinson, J.A., Gibberd, R. & Sanson-Fisher, R.W. (1990a). Accuracy of pap smear self-report: a methodological consideration in cervical screening research, *Health services research*, in press.

Bowman, J., Redman, S., Reid, A. & Sanson-Fisher, R. (1990b). General practitioners and Pap smear provisions: current practice knowledge and attitudes, *The medical journal of Australia*, 152, 178–183.

Branca, P. (1978). *Women in Europe since 1750*, Croom Helm, London.

Brown, M. (1985). Female infertility — causes, options, priorities and IVF, *Women's health in a changing society*, Proceedings of the 2nd national conference on all aspects of women's health, Adelaide, September, 168–170.

Carmody, D.A. (1985). A positive approach towards adolescent sexuality, *Women's health in a changing society*, vol. 2, Proceedings of the 2nd national conference on all areas of women's health, Adelaide, September.

Chapman, S. & Hodgson, J. (1988). Showers in raincoats: attitudinal barriers to condom use in high-risk heterosexuals, *Community health studies*, 12 (1), 97–105.

Clark, M. (1985). Women's health and sexually transmitted diseases, *Women's health in a changing society*, Proceedings of the 2nd national conference on all aspects of women's health, Adelaide, September, pp 95–97.

Coombs, J. (1985). Abortion: a woman's right? *Women' s health in a changing society*, vol. 2, Proceedings of the 2nd national conference on all areas of women's health, Adelaide, September, p. 99.

Daniel, A. (1985). NSW health care and discretionary surgery statistics, *The medical journal of Australia*, 142, 251–253.

Dicker, R.G., Greenspan, J.R., Strauss, L.T., Cowart, M.R., Scally, M.J., Peterson, H.B., DeStefano, F., Rubin, G.L. & Ory, H.W. (1982). Complications of abdominal and vaginal hysterectomy among women of reproductive age in the United States, *American journal of obstetrics and gynaecology*, 144, 841–8.

Dickinson, J.A., Leeder, S.R. & Sanson-Fisher, R.W. (1988). Frequency of cervical smear-tests among patients of general practitioners, *The medical journal of Australia*, 148, 128–131.

Douglas, F., Greenoff, J. & Woodroffe, S. (1984–6). Chlamidyal infection in women, *Annual report of the Menzies school of health research*, July 1984–June 1986, 65–66.

Easterday, C.L., Grimes, D.A. & Riggs, J.A. (1983). Hysterectomy in the United States, *Obstetrics and gynaecology*, 62 (3), 203–212.

Enkin, M. & Chalmers, I. (1982). *Effectiveness and satisfaction in antenatal care*, William Heinemann, London.

Fleming, W.B. (1985). The cancer-related check-up: a guide for medical practitioners, *The medical journal of Australia*, 143, 33–40.

Fraser, I.S. (1988). Non-oral hormonal contraceptives — the way to the future? *Patient management*, 12 (7), 77–87.

Furstenburg, F.F., Brooks-Gunn, J.J. & Chase-Lansdale, L. (1989). Teenage pregnancy and childbearing, *American psychologist*, 214, 313–320.

Garland, S.M. & Johnson, B. (1989). Chlamydia trachomatis infections — the Royal Women's Hospital experience, *The medical journal of Australia*, 150, 174–177.

Gilbert, G.L. (1987). Treatment of chlamydial and mycoplasmal genital infection, *The medical journal of Australia*, 146, 205–207.

Hakama, M., Chamberlain, L., Day, N.E., Miller, A.B. & Prorok, P.C. (1985). Evaluation of screening programs for gynaecological cancer, *British journal of cancer*, 52, 669–673.

Harrison, S.M. (1985). New perspectives in minimising the physical effects of childbearing, *Women's health in a changing society*, Proceedings of the 2nd national conference on all aspects of women's health, Adelaide, September, pp 168–170.

Holmes, B. (1985). The consequences of unplanned pregnancy — an overview, *Women's health in a changing society*, Proceedings of the 2nd national conference on all aspects of women's health, Adelaide, September, pp 207–216.

Holmes, H.B., Hoskings, B. & Gross, M. (eds) (1980). *Birth control and controlling birth: women centred perspectives*, The Humana Press, Clifton NJ.

Hulka, B. (1982). Risk factors for cervical cancer, *Journal of chronic diseases*, 35, 3–11.

Hurse, E. (1985). Abortion — the Queensland situation, *Women's health in a changing society*, proceedings of the 2nd national conference on all aspects of women's health, Adelaide, September, pp 216–219.

Illich, I. (1976). *Medical nemesis*, Pantheon, New York.

Jones, E.F. (1985). Teenage pregnancy in developed countries: determinants and policy implications, *Family planning perspectives*, 17 (2), 53–63.

Khoo, S.K. (1989). Contraceptive efficacy of the Pill, *The medical journal of Australia*, 150, 548–549.

Kovacs, G.T., Westcott, M., Rusden, J. (1988). Microbiological profile of the cervix in 1000 sexually active women, *Australia and New Zealand journal of obstetrics and gynaecology*, 28 (3), 216–220.

Kovacs, G.T., Riddoch, G., Duncombe, P., Welberry, L., Chick, P., Weisberg, E., Leavelsy, G.M. and Baker, H.W.G. (1989). Inadvertent pregnancies in oral contraceptive users, *The medical journal of Australia*, 150, 549–551.

Lennane, K.J. & Lennane, R.J. (1973). Alleged psychogenic disorders in women — a possible manifestation of several prejudices, *New England journal of medicine*, 288, 288–292.

Lewin, E. & Olesen, V. (1985). *Women, health and healing*, Tavistock: New York.

Llewellyn-Jones, D. (1986). *Fundamentals of obstetrics and gynaecology*, vol. I, 4th edition, Faber and Faber, London.

Maternity services in NSW (1989). *Final report of the Ministerial taskforce on obstetric services in NSW*, January, New South Wales Department of Health, Sydney.

Mitchell, H. & Medley, G. (1987). Age trends in pap smear usage 1971–86, *Community health studies*, vol. 11, 183–5.

Mitchell, J. & Oakley, A. (1976). *The rights and wrongs of women*, Penguin books, London.

NH & MRC (1988a). *Report on maternal deaths in Australia 1982–1984*, June.

NH & MRC working party report (1988b). *Pelvic inflammatory disease*, November.

National women's health policy (1989). *National women's health policy: advancing women's health in Australia*, AGPS, Canberra.

Neefus, M. & Taylor, M. (1981). Educational needs of hysterectomy patients, *Patient counselling and health education*, 3, 150–154.

Office of Population Censuses and Surveys, (1983). *Cancer statistics*, Registrations series MB 12 HMSO London.

Oakley, A. (1982). The origins and development of antenatal care, in Enkin, M. & Chalmers, I. (eds) *Effectiveness and satisfaction in antenatal care*, William Heineman, London.

O'Hara, M.W. (1987). Post partum 'blues', depression and psychosis: a review, *Journal of psychosomatic obstetrics and gynaecology*, 7 (3), 205–227.

O'Hara, M.W., Neuraber, D.J. & Zekoski, E.M. (1984). Prospective study of post partum depression: prevalence, course and predictive factors, *Journal of abnormal psychology*, 93 (2), 159–171.

Paul, C., Skegg, D., Spears, G. & Kaldor, J.M. (1986). Oral contraceptives and breast cancer: a national study, *British medical journal*, 293, 723–726.

Philpot, C.R., Harcourt, C., Edwards, J. & Grealis, A. (1988). Human immunodeficiency virus and female prostitutes, *Genitourinary medicine*, 64 (3), 193–197.

Pohlman, E. (1969). *Psychology of birth planning*, Schenkman, Massachusetts.

Redman, S., Hennrikus, D.J., Bowman, J.A. & Sanson-Fisher, R. (1988). Assessing women's health needs, *The medical journal of Australia*, 148, 123–127.

Report of the Public health service task force on women's health issues vol. 1 (1985). *Public health reports*, 100 (1), 73–105.

Rohan, T.E. & McMichael, A.J.(1977). *Oral contraceptive agents and breast cancer: a population-based case-control study*.

Royal Commission on Human Relationships (1977). *Final report*, AGPS, Canberra.

Russell, J. & Johnson, G.F. (1987). Premenstrual syndrome, *The medical journal of Australia*, 146, 510–511.

Sambrook, P. & Eisman, J. (1989). The clinical management of osteoporosis, *Healthright*, 8 (2), 23–26.

Sandberg, S.I., Barnes, B.A., Weinstein, M.C. & Braun, P. (1985). Elective hysterectomy — benefits, risks and costs, *Medical care*, 23, 1067–1085.

Sexually transmitted disease surveillance (1982). *Weekly epidemiological records*, 57, 220–221.

Schacht, P.J. & Pemberton, A. (1985). What is unnecessary surgery? Who shall decide? Issues of consumer sovereignty, conflict and self-regulation, *Social science in medicine*, 20, 199–206.

Shearman, R.P. (1986). Oral contraceptive agents, *The medical journal of Australia*, 144, 210–204.

Smithurst, B.A. & Armstrong, J.L. (1975). Social background of 171 women attending a female venereal disease clinic in Brisbane, *The medical journal of Australia*, 15, 339–343.

Stanley, F.J. & Straton, J.A.Y. (1981). Teenage pregnancies in Western Australia, *The medical journal of Australia*, 2, 468–469.

WHO Scientific Group (1981). Research on the menopause, *WHO technical report series 670*, WHO, Geneva.

8 Women and Body Image

The image that we call a woman's body has both societal and individual components. The individual factors include, the physical self which relates to the genetic make up and biological expression, personal decisions women make about their body shape, women's responses to their food intake and related disorders and the clinical response to these disorders. The societal factors include society's perception of women which has class, race, and economic constituents. The way society chooses to view women can have profound effects on the way women view themselves. Acceptable body images, stereotyping of women, traditional role expectations, and the feminist view of these influences, all contribute to the continuing conflicts women have in relation to the way they view themselves.

VISIONS OF WOMEN

Women of the 15th and 16th century are depicted by such artists as Titian, Giorgiones, Michaelango and Raphael as well endowed, perhaps 70 kilograms in weight. They are usually naked, plump, pink, vulnerable, passive, either sexually submissive or maternally nurturing. In viewing the post-war images of Australian women through such magazines as *The Australian Women's Weekly*, the image of the 1940s woman is not so different from her predecessor of 500 years before, except that she is now fully clothed and ten kilograms lighter, entirely house-bound and particularly interested in feeding the family and keeping her home shiny and clean. The glossy magazines of the 1980s and 1990s show the ideal woman as weighing approximately 50 kilograms. She has dropped ten kilograms in one generation compared with the ten kilograms she lost in the previous 500 years. She often manages a full-time career, but is just as devoted to feeding her husband and children as ever before, albeit with a new scientific precision.

WOMEN AND THE MEDIA

Women are frequently reminded of the ideal body type by media, advertising and health care professionals. Garner et al. (1980) reviewed images of women in magazine articles for 20 years between 1960 and 1980 and demonstrated that the average weight for height decreased significantly over the period. The weights of many of these women appeared to be below the average weight of American women. In reviewing the same journals, Garner found a significant increase in the number of diet articles appearing. On average each magazine published four diet articles per year. Whilst journals continue to focus on the ideal woman, women consumers are more sceptical of this view. Crawford and Worsley's (1988) study of South Australian women found that 90 per cent of women who were surveyed believed that magazines should not make such an issue of slimness.

In addition to the women's magazine industry, there are billion dollar medical, pharmaceutical and weight reduction industries dependent on the preservation of the concept of the ideal woman as slim. Health care professionals also pressure women to lose weight. Ashwell (1973) and Yudkin (1973) report that overweight women are treated more aggressively by medical practitioners than overweight men.

In recent times, whilst advertising and other media messages convey 'positive' images of women, the individual life experiences of women are often contrary. Through sexual discrimination and sexual harassment in the workplace, through contradictory messages from childhood about women's social role, and aided by pornography and 'put downs', many women have lost confidence in their perceptions of their bodies. For example, advertisements on television and elsewhere show slim, supposedly healthy women engaging in activities which can be envied by viewers. However, few viewers will be as 'perfect' as these 'television' women who have been selected on the basis of how well they portray an ideal — an ideal usually created by male advertising executives.

Body image refers to a woman's perception of her body. Schilder (1935) defines body image as the picture of our own body which we form in our mind. It is not just a mental reflection of the physical self but is partly formed by other people's appraisals of and reactions to our appearance and actions. This view is not necessarily consistent with actual physical appearance. Simmons and Rosenberg (1975) and Lerner, Orlos and Knapp (1976) suggest that body image makes a greater contribution to self esteem in women than in men. Rodin, Silberstein and Striegel-Moore (1985) add that women also tend to be less satisfied with their body.

BODY IMAGE IN ADOLESCENCE

Adolescent girls are confronted by the need for effective decision making regarding their health and lifestyle practices at a time of rapid personal development.

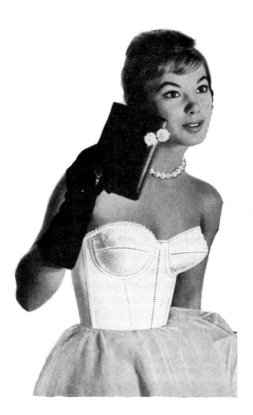

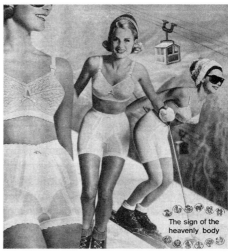

The sign of the
heavenly body

1964

*From the 1940s to the 1990s, magazine images
of women demonstrate that the average
weight for height decreased significantly —
ten kilograms were lost in one generation,
compared with the ten kilograms lost over the
previous 500 years*

1959

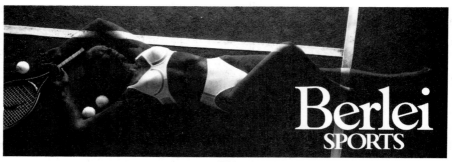

Berlei
SPORTS

1990

Peterson and Brooks-Gunn (1988) assert that adolescence is a time of high risk for girls. It is unmatched throughout their life span. Girls are experimenting with independence, exploring sexuality, acquiring new skills, e.g. driving, engaging in competitive sports and testing at-risk behaviours such as drug and alcohol consumption. For example, Alexander (1980) reports that one in three girls between the ages of 15–19 years is sexually active and ten per cent become pregnant (see chapter seven).

Maturation studies have shown that satisfaction with body decreases as girls pass through puberty. Davies and Furnham (1986) discovered that from age 12–18 years there is a noticeable decline in satisfaction with the body concomitant with the girl's exposure to social and cultural pressures towards assuming a particular body type. During early adolescence, Clifford (1971) suggests, girls become more self conscious, have lower self esteem and express more dissatisfaction with body image. By late adolescence when the body shape of the adolescent girl is formed for adulthood, the relationship between self esteem and satisfaction with physical attractiveness in girls is completed.

Girls perceive their bodies as out of control in adolescence. The sudden increase in body fat is frightening in the context of powerful social constraints against fatness. One theory suggests that in order to gain control over their bodies within these social constraints, girls compete with other girls to make themselves less fat, in the process making themselves smaller and skinnier and less physically powerful. Quadrio (1983) calls this the 'paradoxical bind' where girls compete not by becoming physically and emotionally stronger but rather by becoming smaller, weaker and sexually passive and thus attempt to win control over their bodies, status and acceptability in their peer group by losing physical power.

There are no Australian data on the changing notions on body image in specific cultural groups of adolescent girls. However, groups influenced by the western patterns of advertising, female work/home contradictions, and societal thinness as the normative state would be expected to exhibit these patterns.

Girls not only have to contend with the social and physiological changes of adolescence. Griffith-Kenney (1986) notes that certain health problems of adolescence also contribute adversely to the developing body image of adolescent girls. Conditions affecting facial appearance can contribute to negative body image. Myopia (short-sightedness), astigmatism and other disorders of vision which result in disability or the wearing of glasses are one such group of hindrances. Eighty per cent of adolescent girls are affected by acne which is often viewed by them as a disfiguring condition. The conventional wisdom that diet was a major contributor to the severity of acne meant that girls were placed in a no-win situation where if they did not follow a diet to prevent acne, similar to a weight-loss diet, then acne would be encouraged to the detriment of their self-image. Recent evidence from Michaelson (1981) and others suggest that diet has very little role in the control of acne.

THE IDEAL WOMAN

From an early age women have been traditionally taught that the attractiveness of their body will determine life's success. Much of a woman's status has been derived from her ability to catch and marry a desirable man. Less of her prestige has come from her work or her income. Women are therefore ambivalent about their career success relative to physical attractiveness. They perceive that such success may make them less attractive to men. Orbach (1978) notes that the image formulated of a successful woman is ...

appealing, earthy, sensual, sexual, virginal, innocent, reliable, daring, mysterious, coquettish, and thin.

Our society is very prescriptive about acceptable body types for women. Even pregnant women are not immune. Graham (1976) suggests that they are subjected to images of pregnancy in handbooks on 'mothercare' which tend to romanticise pregnancy and create an image of the pregnant woman at one with nature, serene etc. Regardless of how women actually look, part of their body image will be shaped by the societal ideal of how women should look. The stronger the notion of the ideal body type the more likely it is that an individual will be concerned about her own body.

Quadrio (1983) suggests that today's female stereotype is full of contradiction. The ideal woman continues to be represented as passive, nurturing, home centred, and a sexual object and yet she is also depicted as outgoing, assertive and sexually active. Barrett and Roberts (1978) in their study of British general practitioners identified the contributory role the medical profession plays in supporting these contradictions. Whilst advising middle-aged women with grown up children to look for part-time jobs, the same general practitioners would advise them to give up the work at the first sign of personal or family dysfunction caused by the altered roles and lifestyle expectations, rather than look at ways in which the family as a whole could tackle the problems.

In the patterns established in adolescence in western society, the ideal body for women is slim. It is physically disempowering for women to lose too much weight as it renders them more likely to also lose 'female' hormones which contribute to the female look, visually distinguishing women from men. In addition, significantly less than optimal weight contributes to infertility by decreasing the likelihood of ovulation and thereby diminishing women's power to control procreation (see chapter seven). Lost in the western world is the 'Rubenesque' view of women current during the seventeenth century which continued until the end of the Victorian era and celebrated the feminine, childbearing, nurturing form.

Her face is round ... her shoulders softly rounded ... her bosom, in its luxuriances, seems literally to protrude on the space occupied by her arms ... her thighs are large in proportion ... the whole figure is soft and voluptuous in the extreme ... excessive leanness is repulsive ... (Reichman 1977).

Advertising has inflicted on women, particularly young women, messages which are not only mixed, but which are mutually exclusive and unable to be pieced together in a coherent framework. Add to this the conflicts young women feel when they see their images objectified in these advertisements and it is not surprising that they have difficulty co-ordinating their psychological and physical images of themselves.

The qualities endowed by female anthromorphism and female sex hormones and their implications for fertility are respected and revered in other cultures. For example in some South Pacific cultures, obesity in women is encouraged. In these cultures, and indeed in all cultures, female hormones, oestrogen and progesterone are believed to offer a protective effect against the negative consequence of obesity. In the Pacific Basin, for example the development of non-insulin dependent diabetes is more common amongst obese men than women.

Today's ideal woman should be young. Mature women are by definition unattractive and all signs of ageing should be disguised. In their study of women attending general practitioners, Barrett and Roberts (1978) found that middle-aged

Consumer watchdog rips into skin 'repair' cosmetics

'Anti-aging' cosmetics that sell for up to $270 for a tiny 30-gram jar are little more than glorified moisturisers, according to the consumer magazine, *Choice*.

The May issue of the magazine dashes the hopes of consumers who have trusted claims that such creams can 'repair' and 'rebuild' aging skin.

'The most blatant fallacy included in advertisements for these cosmetics is that because they contain ingredients that occur naturally in the body like collagen and elastin, they can directly replenish the body's supply of these proteins.

'As a crude analogy, eating bone would not repair a broken arm, so putting 'soluble' elastin or collagen on your face won't repair or restructure saggy skin.'

The Australian Consumers' Association, which publishes *Choice*, has called for marketers of products which make therapeutic claims to be forced either to register the product as a drug, drop the claims or withdraw the product.

Dr Alan Cooper, honorary secretary of the Australian College of Dermatologists, said yesterday that he supported and endorsed the *Choice* report.

'If something is penetrating the skin, causing physiological changes, it is a drug and should be meeting a whole series of strict guidelines for drugs,' Dr Cooper said.

'If it is not, its makers should not be making therapeutic claims.'

In the wake of complaints about therapeutic claims for cosmetics in advertisements, the Commonwealth Department of Community Services and Health has written to some cosmetic companies asking them to drop their claims.

Mr John Majewsky, the managing director of Narhex, which markets the product Cross-Linked 10/60 Elastin, said yesterday that Narhex had not received such a letter.

Narhex uses a prominent media personality, Ms Ita Buttrose, and the slogan 'Science To Slow Aging' in its print advertisement.

However, Mr Geoffrey Dutton, the head of the advertising of therapeutic goods section in the Department of Health, said Narhex had been told two years ago, in relation to its planned television advertising, that the slogan and therapeutic claims were not acceptable.

Narhex confirmed the slogan and claims had not been used in its subsequent television commercials.

Mr Dutton said Narhex had not been sent the more recent warning letter 'because no complaints have been received about its print ads.'

The introduction of the *Therapeutic Goods Act*, delayed because of the election, should lead to tighter regulations, *Choice* says.

Miss Judith Myers, Helena Rubinstein's product manager for 'Intercell — The first all-round anti-aging Gel Cream' said: 'Until the act is in force and they tell us exactly what we can and can't say, our advertising will stay the same.'

Choice's advice to consumers on the best strategies to combat aging? Wear a hat and a sunscreen.

Meryl Constance, *Sydney Morning Herald*, 15 May 1990

women were more likely to receive psychotropic drugs (see chapter ten), be advised to take part-time jobs, and more likely to be described in terms of their families than women of other ages and men in general. It is also less than ideal to have body hair or smells, or be untanned, if the plethora of commercial preparations available to deal with these tragedies is any indication.

HEALTH CONSEQUENCES

Throughout history there have been examples of negative health consequences from pressure on women to assume a particular body shape. One of the best known is foot binding of girl babies in China. Designed to achieve small and beautiful feet, this process crippled many women.

Australian contemporary society also has many examples, e.g. hair dyes containing phenylenediamines and toluenediamines are suspected of being carcinogenic. Surgery to change the shape of breasts can result in damage to the sensory nerves leading to the nipple. Morgrave (1985) believes that between 10 and 40 per cent of women undergoing this surgery end up with painful, swollen and distorted breasts. In 1982, Llewellyn-Jones dispelled the myths about vaginal odour and identified the medical consequences of use of vaginal deodorants, including allergic inflammation and infection.

The promotion of tanned skin as attractive has probably been responsible for many deaths from skin cancer, particularly amongst women whose skin is naturally fair. There is considerable debate as to whether high-heeled shoes are health hazards. Podiatrists are united in describing the damaging effects on posture and foot care. Orthopaedic surgeons are divided in their opinions as to whether the body adjusts or not.

WEIGHT

Traditional methods for assessing weight have been based on tables derived from American life insurance data collected in 1959. As few women worked in 1959 and therefore took out life insurance, this measure of women's weight has been inappropriate. In an effort to develop a less culturally bound measure the Body Mass Index (BMI) was introduced. This measurement takes into account a woman's weight and height to form a ratio which is compared with a pre-established norm. As the pursuit of thinness has been a dominant feature of women's health over the latter part of the century, any standardised benchmark for women developed during this time is of questionable significance. Based on the BMI, the *National Heart Foundation risk factor prevalence study* (1983) found that eight per cent of women were able to be classified as obese. Twenty-six per cent of the study population of women were found to be overweight.

In evaluating the proportion of women who are overweight it is important to distinguish between being overweight in terms of societal attractiveness and being overweight in health terms. Recently the societal view that women should be slim to be attractive has been given face validity by the health movement which has pointed out the potentially harmful effects of obesity. The relationship between obesity and increased mortality from cancer, cardiovascular disease, and diabetes has been well documented. However, the relationship between being overweight and poor health has not been established   Using the National Heart Foundation figures, only eight per cent of women can be considered to have a serious health risk on account of their weight.

Although most women are within a health weight range, a study by Redman et al. (1988) of Australian women reported that 50 per cent of women were concerned about their weight. In Crawford and Worsley's study 38 per cent of the women indicated that they had dieted in the previous year, 15 per cent had fasted, 10 per cent had taken slimming tablets, 6 per cent had used diuretic agents, and 3 per cent had used laxative agents to control their weight. Abraham (1983) estimates that up to 20 per cent of young women may fulfil the criteria for an eating disorder at some time. Women are more aware of obesity both in others and in themselves (Worsley 1981; Miller et al. 1980). They express more desire to lose weight and more concern over body weight and are more likely than men to believe they are overweight (Dwyer and Mayer 1970; Jeffrey et al. 1984). Women weigh themselves more frequently than men and conclude more often that reducing is necessary even though their weight may be within normal range. These findings are also supported by the National Heart Foundation data and the Newcastle studies of Redman et al.

SELF ESTEEM

A concern about being overweight has a damaging effect on self esteem. Wooley, Wooley and Dyrenforth (1979) say that stereotyping of obese people begins in childhood with girls rating obese girls as being more lazy, ugly, dishonest, sloppy, mean and dirty. By early adulthood obese women are viewed as self pitying, obnoxious and far more frequently anxious than normal weight women according to Waldroop (1980). Obesity has been shown to be the least preferred physical characteristic for girls to possess even when physical handicaps are included in the choices. The passive victim role of being handicapped is more appealing to women than the difficult and ambivalent task of controlling their weight. Whilst in most cases women are not obese they continue to attribute these negative stereotypes to themselves and therefore suffer under the consequent reduction in self esteem.

DIETING

At any given time, Crawford and Worsley extrapolate, more than 30 per cent of Australian women will be undertaking weight loss diets. There are a plethora of organisations helping women to lose weight. In her review of self-help groups and for-profit weight loss organisations in Australia, Levy et al. (1986) highlights that they are attended almost exclusively by women the majority of whom are of normal or less than normal weight. Many women believe that dieting can work if only enough will power is applied. Levy showed that attenders at self help groups for weight loss were able to achieve an average loss of only four kilograms over a 17 week program. Long term reviews of dieting programs conclude that most obese women regain the weight they lost during treatment over the 12 months following the end of treatment. Similarly, weight loss programs have a high drop out rate. Volkmer et al. (1981) cites the Weight Watchers program as an example: 70 per cent will leave the program within three months and 90 per cent by 12 months. Drop outs are generally assumed to have left the program because they are not succeeding. The process of dieting and the inevitable failure to lose weight will have a negative effect on a woman. She already feels inadequate because she perceives herself as being overweight, her failure to diet successfully reinforces her view of herself as lacking in self control.

There are also physiological effects of dieting. Restricting calories can maintain an obese state as this process also slows down the metabolic rate. A low calorie diet may also make the woman too tired to exercise and therefore expend calories. Bray (1976) has shown that dietary restriction puts stress on the cardiovascular system and can increase the negative effects of cholesterol. Thus the natural advantage in relation to cholesterol provided to women in oestrogen can be lost through dieting. In young women, dieting has been associated with amenorrhea, depression, and impaired ability to perform in school. Wooley goes further to suggest that fluctuations in weight from dieting are more damaging to women's health than being consistently overweight.

ANOREXIA NERVOSA AND BULIMIA

Anorexia nervosa and related syndromes involve voluntary resistance to eating, often accompanied by laxative abuse and induced vomiting and therefore characterised by excessive self induced weight loss. The woman's weight may be as much as 50 per cent below normal. It is usually found in adolescent girls and young women (90 per cent). Anorexia nervosa is usually first seen between the ages of 15 and 20. In Australia it has been estimated that one in sixteen schoolgirls are anorexic. Classic symptoms of anorexia nervosa are resistance to eating, loss of body weight, amenorrhoea, low blood pressure and biochemical imbalances. Kalucy (1983) estimates that it is associated with a mortality risk of between 10 and 20 per cent in the absence of treatment. Because anorexic young women frequently deny they are starving themselves they are often treated inappropriately for problems secondary to anorexia nervosa, such as amenorrhoea, cyclical oedema, osteoporosis, unexplained weight loss, Raynaud's disease, and thyroid disorders.

The over estimation of body size which occurs in both women of normal weight and obese women is more pronounced amongst women with anorexia nervosa. Slade and Russell (1973) found that women suffering from anorexia nervosa over estimated their body size by between 27 and 58 per cent. During treatment, weight gain led to an increase in real size and these patients became more accurate in their assessments of their weight. Treatment methods include psychotherapy, behaviour modification, traditional physical support and family therapy. Unfortunately, Fogel and Woods (1981) believe that no single specific treatment is successful on a long term basis.

Although there are several theories accounting for the development of anorexia the most influential has been based on the argument that anorexic young women have a disordered body image. They believe they are overweight when in fact they are not. Typically the anorexic girl comes from a background of high expectations.

Bulimia is another eating disorder characterised by current episodes of binge eating. Potts (1984) estimated that between 15 and 20 per cent of American college women prevent weight gain by a 'binge-and-purge' eating style. These binges induce feelings of guilt in the bulimic girl which force her to purge herself by vomiting or taking purgatives. Binge-eating usually occurs daily in the active

New study finds anorexia causes brain damage

Slimmers who fall victim to anorexia nervosa risk permanent brain damage, new research has revealed.

Although modern medicine has managed to stop most anorexia sufferers from dying, doctors are now finding that many of those who survive are left with serious, probably incurable changes in their brain structure.

Writing in the *British Medical Journal*, Dr George Patton, a lecturer in psychiatry at the Royal Free Hospital, London, said brain scans of anorexic patients had 'shown structural changes to the brain' and 'weight gain does not reverse' those changes.

The parts of the brain affected are the grooves between the lobes of the brain (which got wider) and the spaces holding the fluid which bathes the brain (which got larger).

Researchers believe the reason for these changes might be loss of brain tissue due to chronic starvation.

Post-mortems on anorexia nervosa victims have found evidence of destruction in the areas of the brain responsible for higher functions like thinking and talking.

Anorexics are often highly intelligent over achievers, but doctors at the Royal Free Hospital have seen some of their patients deteriorate quite noticeably.

One young man patient was unable to walk or talk — at first they thought his problem was psychological but later realised it was at least partly due to brain damage.

Although most researchers believe the brain damage seen in anorexia nervosa is caused by chronic lack of necessary nutrients, some say it might possibly be due to brain damage at birth.

A large number of anorexics suffered complications at birth and birth complications can lead to the kind of brain damage seen in anorexia nervosa.

The brain isn't the only part of the body damaged by anorexia nervosa. The bones also become seriously weakened because the body takes the calcium it needs from the bones when there is not enough in the daily diet.

This problem, osteoporosis, is reversible and most anorexics' bones recover when they go back to a normal eating pattern, but those who still keep their weight low commonly break their bones without falling or stressing them in any significant way.

Despite the disastrous consequences of anorexia nervosa, doctors are actually getting better at treating it — or at least preventing its ultimate consequence: death.

Thirty years ago at least three in 20 anorexics died. Now the figure is closer to one in 30.

However, though in the past most were dying from starvation, these days half the anorexics who die take overdoses — which suggests they were determined to die one way or another.

And while the rate of death in the early years of the disease has dropped, getting an anorexic over the initial phases is only part of the battle.

Recent long-term studies have shown that anorexics are likely to die from the disease years after they are first diagnosed as suffering from it.

Those people who don't return to a normal weight and eating habits are likely to die from the disease as long as 20 years after first seeing a doctor for the problem.

However, not all people who get anorexia are doomed to irreversible brain damage, broken bones and an early death.

A study in Sweden found that a quarter of patients recover within three years, half after six years and 75 per cent after 12 years.

Margaret Harris, *Sun-Herald*, 23 July 1989.

phase. Foster (1985) reports that in one study of 40 women the mean number of episodes per week was 12. The duration of the eating period could last up to eight hours and the amount of food ingested could be up to 50,000 calories a day.

Disordered body image may also contribute to bulimia. Women with bulimia over estimate their body widths but can accurately judge a neutral object. This condition is another result of the conflicting pressures placed on adolescent women.

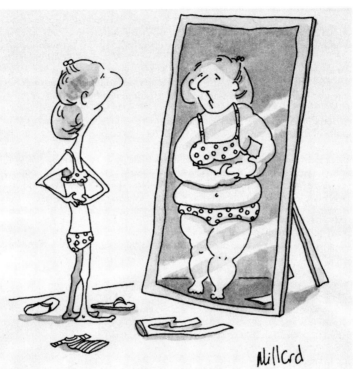

WOMEN AND PORNOGRAPHY

Another influence detrimental to a woman's search for a valid self image is the publication of so-called soft-core pornography, such as *Playboy*, *Penthouse* and *Hustler*. By socialising the view of women as unreal sex objects, *Playboy* and the magazines which follow its lead have contributed to the increasing antagonism between males and females as to the appropriate portrayal of sex scenes. Women are portrayed in these magazines as powerless and subservient. These images usually confirm women as passive, fetished objects for male consumption. Some feminists suggest that the implied violence can incite men into sexually violent acts against women. Opponents of this argument suggest that sexual violence would not decrease if pornography was banned as the underlying cause of this violence, i.e. male hostility towards women remains. They suggest that this extreme position polarises images of men and women and prohibits healthy exploration of sexual imagery.

More recently women have attempted to separate the punitive and negative aspects of pornographic visions from the more woman sensitive notion of erotica. However, in this process a new type of sexual subservience is created. Willis (1984) suggests that the view of sex that most often emerges from talk about erotica is sentimental and euphemistic. She argues that this concept of eroticism is not feminist but feminine. In order to reclaim pornography, distinctions must be made between forms of pornography which are women sensitive and those that incite violence against women and children and perpetuate stereotyping of women.

The factions within the women's movement are exemplified by the pornography debate. The feminism of the 1960s which was characterised by a belief in a social construction of gender and an emphasis of the elimination of gender difference polarised this group's opinions about pornography. Men were not seen as oppressors because of their male biology but rather because of their rationalisation of their supremacy based on male biology. Pornography was seen to validate this position by reinforcing the male power to visually subjugate women.

A more recent view of women's oppression as developing from a repression of female values has given rise to the cultural feminist movement. This group is characterised by a belief that reclaiming and celebrating the female identity would be the solution to patriarchal oppression. Equally strong in their anti-pornographic stance, this group polarised sexuality into women's sexuality which was seen as loving, sensuous and spiritual whilst men's sexuality was seen as genitally orientated, compulsive and violent.

An assumption of the anti-pornography critique is that pornographic images do not (and should not) give pleasure to women. Coward (1987) highlights the contradiction this holds for women:

> this appears to reverse the previous commitment in feminist politics, to the positive assertion of women's active and independent sexual needs, whether they be with men or women.

Willis (1984) goes further to suggest that pornography is used as a way for women to oppress other women, for example, by saying 'what turns me on is erotic; what turns you on is pornographic'.

Another criticism of the anti-pornography stance is that the rejection of sexual permissiveness connects it to other oppressive and extremist views often expressed in the Right. Echols (1984) highlights this:

> the cultural feminist solution to male lasciviousness is the reestablishment of old-fashioned respect, which the sexual revolution has destroyed. This analysis confuses respect with equality and fails to recognize that respect is merely the flip side of violation. More importantly, this view suggests that sexual repression is a satisfactory solution to the real problem of violence against women.

Willis (1984) supports Echols' view that the relationship between pornography and violence is not causative. She points out that most pornography by definition is overtly sexual and not violent. At this point the differentiation between violent pornography and non-violent pornography, often now equated with erotica, becomes necessary. Other factors need to be explored in developing a broad based

approach to pornography. Class, race and sexual preference are only now beginning to enter the discussion.

CASE STUDY

Jessie had been to the Young People's Resource Centre four times now, and wondered why
it had such a formal name, when it was such an easy place to feel at home. Tonight she was
going to go to Dot's discussion group again; her friend Sally had taken her for the first time
two weeks ago. They didn't quite know why they liked the discussions — which were basically about feeling good about how you look. Somehow they seemed to answer some of the
questions Jessie and her friends had, even before they had got around to putting them into
words.

By the time the discussion started there were eight in the group — all between thirteen
and sixteen — and the leader, Dot, who was a clinical psychologist working at the centre.

They talked a bit about how they felt about themselves and their bodies, at home and at
school, when they felt confident and when they felt scared.

For the first time Sandy talked about her illness. Sandy was sixteen, and had spent much
of the past year in hospital with anorexia nervosa. It was Dot who had helped her most, so
she still wanted to come to her discussions to be reassured that she could cope with the
scary feelings, and the fears which were almost but not entirely gone. Sandy's parents had
been determined that Sandy was going to 'do something' with her life, and wanted her to
excel at everything she tried. The trouble was that Sandy felt she could never measure up to
their expectations. This had worried her more and more, and at the same time they began to
pressure her about the weight she was losing. Being thin became more and more important,
in fact it became an obsession, and it wasn't until she had talked through how she felt about
her body and her self that she could see that her preoccupation with her weight was part of
a larger issue — how she felt about herself and about the way others saw her.

Even after hours of counselling with Dot it seemed that she had agonised over her weight,
and her eating for so long, that just understanding the causes for her fears did not help much.
It seemed as if the process of 'shall I, shan't I?' seemed to have gained a life of its own, with
or without an underlying problem.

What was funny was that Jessie and one other girl in the group shared the same feelings,
much of their thinking revolved around food, and what they should and shouldn't eat. The
other girl was somewhat overweight, but Jessie was of average build and average weight
and the others in the group couldn't understand how someone like that could spend so
much time agonising about food, and what to eat and what not to eat.

Dot explained to them that the eating is only a means to an end, and Jessie was experiencing the same feelings that many teenagers share. For the first time they were aware
that the way they look, dress, walk, do their hair, and act, carries messages to others about
their personality and lifestyle. That is, their body image was being read by others. Jessie was
not sure what kind of messages she wanted to give to the world about her personality and
her lifestyle, and was scared about dealing with people especially when men looked at her
as if she was attractive to them. That is, the image others were seeing did not always tie in
with the image that Jessie wanted to project. On the days she wanted to hide, she ate more
and wanted to lose her attractiveness. But no sooner had that happened than she wanted to
slim, and would not eat anything much the next day.

Dot explained that after a while the process of whether to eat or not eat became as important as the underlying issues, of being a 'together' person both in one's body and one's mind.
Therefore the problems of all three young women were similar — no matter what their weights
were, they were all absorbed by not being able to coordinate their new physical images with their
new psychological identities. Dot explained that her job was to help them sort out the conflicting

messages they were receiving from the world around them. Advertisements espoused one image which was different from what their parents wanted, and the school promoted something different again, let alone friends, and brothers and sisters. Dot said that young women in their early teenage years in countries such as Australia were having real difficulties sorting all these things out, and it was being reflected in the number of young women who gained excess weight for the first time in their lives, or who lost weight and suffered from anorexia nervosa.

Again Jessie was glad she had come, and felt confident that she had time to explore her own identity, and work out the kind of body image she would have as a young woman....

REFERENCES

Abraham, S., Mira, M., Beaumont, P., Souerbutts, T.D. & Llewellyn-Jones, D. (1983). Eating behaviours among young women, *The medical journal of Australia*, 139, 225–228.

Alexander, A. (1980). Challenge of the 80's, *Journal of school health*, 50, 47.

Ashwell, M.A. (1973). A survey of patients' views of doctors' treatment of obesity, *The practitioner*, 211, 653–58.

Barrett, M. & Roberts, H. (1978). Doctors and their patients in Smart, C. & Smart, B. (eds), *Women, sexuality and social control*, Routledge & Keagan Paul, London.

Bray, G. (1976). *The obese patient*, W.B. Saunders, Philadelphia.

Clifford, E. (1971). Body satisfaction in adolescence, *Perceptual and motor skills*, 33, 119–25.

Coward, R. (1987). Sexual violence and sexuality, *Feminist review*, 309.

Crawford, D. & Worsley, A. (1988). Dieting and slimming practices of South Australian women, *The medical journal of Australia*, 148, 325–31.

Davies, E. & Furnham, A. (1986). Body satisfaction in adolescent girls, *British journal of medical psychology*, 59, 279–87.

Dwyer, J.T. & Mayer, J. (1970). Potential dieters: who are they? *Journal of the American Dietetic Association*, 56, 510–514.

Echols, A. (1984). The new feminism of yin and yang, in Snitnow, E. (ed.) *Desire: the politics of sexuality*, Virago, London.

Fogel, C.I. & Woods, N.F. (eds) (1981). *Health care of women*, Mosby, St. Louis.

Foster, D.W. (1985). Eating disorders: obesity and anorexia nervosa, in Wilson, J.D. & Foster, D.W. (eds), *Williams textbook of endocrinology*, W.B. Saunders, Philadelphia.

Garner, D., Garfinkel, P., Schwartz, D. & Thompson, M. (1980). Cultural expectations of thinness in women, *Psychological reports*, 47, 483–91.

Graham, H. (1976) Images of pregnancy in ante-natal literature, in Smart, C. & Smart, B. (eds) *Women, sexuality and social control*, Routledge & Keagan Paul, London.

Griffith-Kenney, J.W. (1986). *A contemporary women's health*, Addison-Wesley, California.

Jeffrey, R.W., Folsom, A.R., Jacobs, D.R., Gillum, R.E., Taylor, H.L. & Blackburn, H. (1984). Prevalence of overweight and weight-loss behaviour in a metropolitan adult population, the Minnesota Heart Survey experience, *American journal of public health*, 74, 349–352.

Kalucy, R.S. (1983). Eating disorders in young women, *The medical journal of Australia*, 139, 205–206.

Lerner, R., Orlos, J. & Knapp, J. (1976). Physical attractiveness, physical effectiveness and self concept in late adolescents, *Adolescence*, 11, 311–26.

Levy, S., Pierce, J., Denbecki, N. & Cripps, A. (1986). Self help group behavioural treatment for obesity, *The medical journal of Australia*, 145, 436–38.

Llewellyn-Jones, D. (1982). *Everywoman: a gynaecological guide for life*, Faber and Faber, London.

Michaelson, G. (1981). Diet and acne, *Nutrition review*, 39, 105.

Miller, T.M., Coffman, J.G. & Linke, R.A. (1980). Survey on body image, weight and diet of college students, *Journal of the American Dietetic Association*, 77, 561–566.

Morgrave, C. (1985). *Cosmetic surgery*, Penguin, London.

National Heart Foundation (1983). *A profile of Australians, a summary of the National Heart Foundation risk factor prevalence study*, Report No. 2.

Orbach, S. (1978). *Fat is a feminist issue*, Berkely Publishing, New York.

Peterson, A.C. & Brooks-Gunn, T. (1988). Puberty and adolescence, in Blechman, E.A. & Brownell, K.D. (eds) *Handbook of behavioural medicine for women*, (pp. 12–27), Pergammon Press, New York.

Potts, N.L. (1984). Eating disorders — the secret pattern of binge/purge, *American journal of nursing*, 84, 32–35.

Quadrio, C. (1983). Anorexia and agoraphobia, paper presented to the conference *Women in therapy*, ANU, Canberra.

Redman, S., Hennrickus, D., Bowman, J. & Sanson-Fisher, R. (1988). Assessing women's health needs, *The medical journal of Australia*, 148, 123–7.

Reichman, S.T. (1977). *Great big beautiful doll*, Dutton, New York.

Rodin, J., Silberstein, L. & Striegel-Moore, R. (1985). Women and weight: a normative discontent, in Sonderegger, T.B. (ed.) *Psychology and gender: Nebraska symposium on motivation 1985*, (pp. 267–307), University of Nebraska Press, Lincoln.

Schilder, P. (1935). *Image and appearance of the human body*, Keegan, Paul, Trench and Trubner & Co, London.

Simmons, R. & Rosenberg, F. (1975). Sex, sex roles and self image, *Journal of youth and adolescence*, 4, 229–58.

Slade, P.D. & Russell, G.F. (1973). Experimental investigations of bodily perceptions in anorexia nervosa and obesity, *Psychotherapy and psychosomatics*, 22, 359–63.

Volkmer, F.R., Stunkard, A., Woolston, J. & Bailey, R. (1981). High attrition rates in commercial weight reduction programs. *Archives of internal medicine*, 141, 426–428.

Waldroop, J.A. (1980). *Body image, sexual identity and eating disorders*, Paper presented to the American Psychological Association meeting, Montreal, August.

Willis, E. (1984). Feminism, morality and pornography in Snitnow, E. (ed.) *Desire: the politics of sexuality*, Virago, London.

Wooley, O.W., Wooley, S.C. & Dyrenforth, S.R. (1979). Obesity and women: a neglected feminist topic, *Women's studies international quarterly*, 2, 81–92.

Worsley, A. (1981). Teenagers' perceptions of fat and slim people, *International journal of obesity*, 5, 15–24.

Yudkin, J. (1973). Doctors' treatment of obesity, *The practitioner*, 201, 330–35.

9 Women and Mental Health

Women are more often diagnosed as mentally ill and more often treated for their illness with medication. Various theoretical frameworks of mental illness are explored in this chapter, pointing to both individual and gender based social expectations. In practical terms, identification of the variety of health problems defined as mental ill-health and the mismatch of service provision are discussed. The major problems relating to mental health services are the limited access and inappropriate facilities for women.

WHAT IS MEANT BY MENTAL HEALTH?

The Women's Health Services Report (1985) highlights the problem of defining mental health and mental illness. It suggests that definitions of mental illness abound whilst definitions of mental health are more elusive.

Mental health can be considered from two points of view. The individual concept, which identifies the way women think, feel and behave is often expressed in terms of subjective experience, e.g. 'I feel happy/sad' and relates these experiences to state of mind. The Women's Health Services Report (1985) emphasises the importance of acknowledging the individual woman in terms of her mental health. The report expands the perception of a healthy state of mind and relates it to the environment in which women live. Self-acceptance, positive self-esteem, the ability to communicate with and enjoy satisfying relationships with others and freedom from lengthy periods of severe anxiety and depression all become part of the constellation of health.

It is clear that the individual notion cannot explain the wealth of literature which conveys the female experience of mental health and mental health care services. Thus, the second notion of mental health as a collective experience of women which relates to their status in society has developed. Furler (1985) suggests that this latter view, which has been determined by health care providers, the majority of whom are men, prevails. Carmen, Russo and Miller (1981) believe that women collude in the process of defining their mental health in male terms. They argue:

> since men hold the power and authority, women are rewarded for developing a set of psychological characteristics that accommodate to and please men. Such traits — submissiveness, compliance, passivity, helplessness, weakness — have been encouraged in women and incorporated into some prevalent psychological theories in which they are defined as innate or inevitable characteristics of women.

The label as it applies to women implies failure. It is assumed that the woman has not met expectations of her behaviour or has been unable to cope with all the demands placed upon her. This label then acts as a control on other women, who fear being labelled in the same way. It is unfortunate that the medical profession has failed to question whether the expectations or demands that the labelling process confers on women are unreasonable or impossible to meet.

Both Furler and Carmen believe that these 'survival skills' are costly to women. The internalisation of sickness behaviour and its equation with femininity requires the development of complex passive and indirect psychological strategies to endure daily life. The use of active mechanisms for coping with and resolving these conflicts is not always successful. Women are more likely to seek medical help at times of decompensation. Furler suggests that at these times women receive a qualitatively different medical response to mental health problems because the 'male centred' ideas about what is 'healthy' are dominant. The concepts of diagnosis and labelling of illness are integral to this process (see chapters three and five).

Unfortunately, women are trapped between these two approaches. The dissonance between their expectations of themselves, the individual approach and society's definition of what is acceptable to women is often the definition of women's mental health. As Bardwick and Douvan (1971) comment:

> Ambivalence is clearly seen in the simultaneous enjoyment of one's feminine identity, qualities, goals, and achievements and the perception of them as less important, meaningful, or satisfying than those of men.

WHO IS MENTALLY ILL?

The statistics suggest that women are more mentally ill than men. According to the Australian Bureau of Statistics' (1982) *Australian health survey*, 357 000 females and 197 000 men reported mental health problems.

Reynolds (1979) found that 33 per cent of women compared with 20 per cent of men reported emotional problems. The most significant of these problems was depression, both chronic and acute, reported by 16 per cent of the women in the study compared with 7 per cent of the men. In the same year Kupinski and Mackenzie (1979) in their Melbourne study of poverty and mental illness found that chronic depression in women was three times that found in men. Raphael (1984) quotes evidence from hospital admission rates to support her assertion that the incidence of depression, anxiety states, neurotic disorders, affective psychosis and paranoid states that require hospital admission is higher for men than women. Weissman and Kellerman (1977) use data from suicide attempts to suggest that twice as many women suffer from depression as men.

Other disorders of mental health are more common in women. Touyz and Beaumont (1985) assert that women are also far more likely to experience eating disorders. Psychotropic medications are also prescribed in greater numbers for women (see chapter ten). Andrews (1989), in her studies of the Sydney catchment area, has found that agoraphobia is more common in women. There is suggestion that panic attacks and anxiety are also more common in women.

More women complain of psychological symptoms. In analysis of completed general health questionnaires, it has been noted that they complain far more than men of: depression, anxiety, sleeping problems, emotional problems and previous nervous breakdowns. Broverman et al. (1970) quote literature extending back to the early work of Anastasi (1949) as support for their claim that sex role stereotyping affects all such questionnaires. It is also possible that such stereotyping may render the results of such questionnaires invalid. One explanation may be that the compilers of such questionnaires are unable to determine the extent to which they sex-role stereotype. In Broverman's study of clinically trained psychologists, psychiatrists and social workers in the United States, it was found that:

> clinicians are significantly less likely to attribute traits which characterize healthy adults to a woman than they are likely to attribute these traits to a healthy man.

As far as diagnostic labels are concerned, depressions of all kinds, neurosis and psychosomatic disorders are predominantly 'female' disorders. Reynolds and Rizzo (1979) and Lee (1979) found that women report more psychological problems, and more frequently attend general practitioners and psychiatrists than men.

So what do these statistics mean? Are women more prone to mental illness? In order to try to understand the statistics, it is important to understand the theories that have shaped the views expressed by doctors and, more recently, other health care providers.

Until recent times the legitimacy of scientific knowledge has protected from scrutiny the underlying moral assumptions that health care professions make about women's mental health. Rosser (1986) highlights the widely held belief in relation to medical science: 'science describes reality and is presumed "objective"; therefore, the term perspective does not apply to it.' She goes on to show how even the foundations of this belief are now in question:

> With several thousand years of distance, most scientists admit that Aristotle's

experiments, in which he counted fewer teeth in the mouths of women than men, were biased by views that women are inferior to men.

Appropriate platitudes reflecting a change in opinion amongst American psychiatrists in relation to their women patients were expressed over a decade ago by the President of the American Psychiatric Association, Alan Stone, in an address to the annual meeting in 1980:

> As far as I can see, the case against psychiatry as regards women ... requires far more than a minor adjustment of our composite sketch, indeed compels each of us to reexamine not only our theories and therapy but also our own lives and relationships ... Is it possible that ... the questions raised in connection with women touch our personal as well as our professional identity? There can be no new psychology of women that does not require a new psychology of men. That makes necessary a new conception of all our human values and all the paradigms of psychiatry.

It has taken over a decade for these sentiments to be expressed at an Australian psychiatric conference (see box p. 131). Whilst Australian psychiatrists are debating whether their views of women are appropriate, services remain inadequate. In defining future objectives for women's mental health, Thomas (1985) outlined the structural ways in which the current treatment of women's mental health problems is inadequate. Davis and George (1988) go one step further to highlight inadequacies within the consultation process. They suggest that in Australia women's physical symptoms have frequently been explained by doctors as manifestations of psychological problems, so that women appear to report and be diagnosed with a higher incidence of neuroses and depressive psychoses.

The picture, however, is not as clear cut as women centred research suggests. Evers (1985) in her study of single, aged men and women in England noted that, given 'comparable health', men were more likely to be placed in institutional care than women. The only conclusion must be that although women are more likely to be diagnosed as crazy, they can look after themselves better than men and are therefore more likely to remain in their own homes. (see chapter 14). Rather than the negative assumption that institutional care is preferentially given to men, it may be that labelling of mental ill health serves to identify those women who have coping mechanisms which enable them to function outside of institutions. Studies have yet to be conducted to show the positive relationship between the labelling of mental ill health and independent living. The relationship of these issues to the provider-consumer perspective in general is discussed in chapters one and five.

In relation to mental health, the medical profession has codified sexuality and gender behaviour in women, and deemed any variation as sick. Examples of this process are cited by Russo and VandenBos (1980) and include differential rates of prescribing psychotrophic drugs, overservicing for conditions congruent with sex role stereotypes e.g. depression, conversion hysteria and phobias. Certain 'sicknesses' are underserviced, including rape, incest and domestic violence. Smith and David (1975) believe that the lack of objective criteria by which to judge mental illness gives the medical profession free reign in deciding exactly whom to label. Or as Carmen, Russo and Miller (1981) state 'he is assertive whilst she is castrating'. For these women, Smith and David argue, rather than mental illness preceding psychiatric control, the reverse happens.

Female focus has doctors psyched up for congress

Are men and women so different and if so, do they need different models of psychotherapy?

For the first time in 26 years, women and whether their needs are special will be the focus of the Royal Australian and New Zealand College of Psychiatrists' annual congress in Perth next week.

The Resilience of Women in the Face of Adversity will be a theme of interest to the women who make up two-thirds of Australia's psychiatric patients.

But the heated internal debate leading up to the congress, culminating in the college abandoning its original theme *There's nothing sooner dry than a woman's tears*, suggests it will also mark a watershed for the women who account for 40 per cent of the profession in the 1990s.

The battle lines were drawn after the 1988 congress when Dr Carolyn Quadrio, a senior lecturer at the University of NSW, observed in a letter to the college journal that delegates had shown very little interest in papers exploring social issues such as torture, or Aboriginal culture.

She was disappointed, too, that there had not been one female plenary speaker.

'Women represented half of the participants yet not once that week did a female form grace the dais,' she wrote in the December 1988 issue.

In an unusual footnote, the journal's editor, Dr Robert Finlay-Jones, addressed one of Dr Quadrio's 'complaints' with the news that 'leading psychiatrists, of whom the majority are women', were to be invited to Perth in 1990.

The provisional theme of that congress was to be *There's nothing sooner dry than a woman's tears*, a line from John Webster's *The White Devil*, written in the early 17th century.

The June 1989 journal was a sizzling read.

In reply to Dr Quadrio's 'querulous criticisms', Dr Phillip Hamilton, a Melbourne psychiatrist, suggested that she should have applied to present a paper entitled 'Reflections of a Paranoid Anti-narcotherapeutic Feminist on Popular Socialist Themes'.

But another five letters, two of them from men, were wholeheartedly supportive of Dr Quadrio. Some condemned the editor's footnote as 'misogynistic', and 'sarcastic and insulting' and 'smug posturing and paternalistic intellectualism'.

But Dr Finlay-Jones said, in reply, that he had resisted the temptation to label theses comments 'for what they are, which is *ad hominem* remarks, since that would surely provoke another shower of letters about sexist language from those of the sisterhood with a little Latin under their surcingles'.

(Consulting their dictionaries for illumination on a 'surcingle', the respondents found it was 'a girth for a horse or other animal' or a 'girdle with which a garment, especially a cassock, is fastened'.)

Dr Finlay-Jones claimed his actions were both 'constructive and sincere'.

'Firstly, I published Dr Quadrio's letter. Secondly, I tried to choose a theme for the 1990 congress which addressed not just the negative view of women's experiences ... but something more positive, which is that they may be more resilient than men.

'Thirdly, I stated my intention of inviting women to speak on these issues ... in the interests of positive discrimination.'

Women were hardier than men, argued Dr Finlay-Jones, 'getting on with the struggle while men self-piteously turn to the bottle or, the ultimate insult, leap into a premature grave'.

Ruth Dewsbury, *Sydney Morning Herald*, 10 May 1990.

THEORETICAL ISSUES

The basis of mental ill health arises in theories that underpin the very concepts which hold for all relationships in our society: femininity (and masculinity), sexuality and the family. These theories play a significant role in understanding mental health issues for women.

It is interesting to note that stereotyping may be a legacy of the Greeks, as the word 'hysteria' originates from the Greek husterikos, meaning womb. However, documentation of the psychoanalytic position of women has grown out of the work of Sigmund Freud, who developed the theoretical framework of psychoanalysis to look at mental health. His basic assumptions are that the origins of gender differentiation in personality, which occur in the Oedipal period, and developmental tasks of this period, are the ultimate cause of both mental health and neurosis.

There is dispute about the usefulness of Freud's psychoanalytic theory. Freud's (1900) work has been criticised by many because of its essential phallocentricity or, as he puts it in his classic treatise *The interpretation of dreams*, 'in order to simplify my presentation, I shall discuss only the boy's identification with his father.'

His notions of femininity, he admits, are 'unsatisfactory, incomplete and vague'. While acknowledging this weakness in his theory, he attributed the idea of femininity as stemming from the little girl's gradual disappointment in being confronted with anatomical 'deficiency'. Popularised Freudianism certainly uses his concepts of 'penis envy' and 'castration complex' to 'explain' women's inferiority in relation to men.

Much of Freud's original work has been interpreted by psychologists and psychiatrists as providing a definition of femininity and masculinity. In this way, it is the individual, usually the woman, who needs to change or adjust or, indeed, be changed or adjusted, usually by men, rather than the need for change in social conditions.

Until recently therapists have not questioned the sociocultural mores which led Freud to his conclusions. However, Chodorow (1978) suggests that Freud's excesses were only the result of his attempt to describe how women develop in a patriarchal society. Unfortunately, strict adherence to Freud's 'weaknesses' have only served to reinforce notions of the inferiority of women in therapy, by interpreting women's difficulties as failure to achieve true femininity. The therapeutic goal of such therapy is to help women come to terms with their femininity and thus be 'well'.

Mitchell (1975) and the French feminist psychoanalysts take the analysis of Freud's work on psychoanalysis one step further. They see his theories as valid instruments for analysing patriarchy and its effects on women and men. They do not adhere to the notion that his work was essentially descriptive and prescriptive, but rather political in that it allows a closer look at the 'operation of patriarchal law within the life of the individual boy and girl'. Mitchell's (1975) work asserts that the interpretation of Freud's work (rather than Freud's theory), is used to reinforce women's inferior position.

Through the process of reclaiming Freud's theory, concepts such as 'penis-envy' become metaphors for women's striving for equality. This approach requires the metaphorical redefinition of the penis. Rather than a tool of male oppression, the penis is seen as a symbol of power and prestige. Equality also requires a redefinition. The common belief of 'superior' groups is that 'equality' is synonymous with 'sameness'. Such a notion assumes that everyone would like to be the same as them, e.g. that disadvantaged groups such as women want to be the same as 'superior' groups such as men. 'Equality' as it is redefined by Russo refers to the equal right to participate in all areas of the life of society and to pursue one's own potential.

Gender role theories

Chesler (1972) outlines how in the second half of this century views on women as handmaidens to men still pervaded psychoanalytic thought. She quotes Bettleheim, who in Vienna in 1965 summed up the role of women in society thus:

> as much as women want to be good scientists and engineers, they want first and foremost to be womanly companions of men and to be mothers.

Evaluation of roles has provided Bart (1971) with some interesting theories on the genesis of depression in women — particularly in middle-aged women. She believes that depression in the older woman stems from a loss of her self-esteem, which up until then has been intimately attached to herself as wife and mother. With the loss of these roles goes the meaning of life, leaving the woman feeling worthless and useless and often severely depressed. Bart's research showed that the more feminine and traditional the woman (e.g. Jewish mothers), the more common was depression in middle age.

Janeway notes that some women psychiatrists, meanwhile were brave enough to argue about what came first for women: the definition of their function in society or the neurosis. In her work on psychiatry and the women's movement, Janeway states unequivocally that society is the initiator: 'social directives which define feminine gender roles in a limiting and even disabling way, invite a neurotic response'. She goes on to outline how this process of identifying mental illness within the individual and ignoring the societal component has been used with other minorities, e.g. homosexuals:

> The idea that the individual self is innately deviant from the ideals of the culture affects women and male minority groups.

Within the profession of psychology, the majority of practitioners (men) did not even include a discussion of the influences of society on shaping the norms of the mental state, let alone any discussion on which element is the precursor within the framework of their practices. Unfortunately, it was not until the late 20th century that thought on this subject shifted. Calvert (1979) comments on the role of modern psychology :

> psychology is not a neutral science, it is a political ideology defining not only how people should behave, but acting as the agency whereby this definition will be upheld. For women, the ideology commits them to be passive, receptive, conforming, dependent and nurturing. A closer look at these 'feminine' characteristics shows that, while women are socialised to acquire them, these attributes are not actually valued very highly by society.

One of the most destructive aspects of the female gender role attributes is the expectation of passivity rather than action. It can be argued that it is this aspect which is, perhaps, more harmful for women than any of the male gender role expectations are for men. The 'feminine characteristics' are validated only in relation to women's roles as mothers. In the *National women's health policy* (1989) this process is described as 'collapsing':

> Where the health system does focus on women's health needs, it often 'collapses' a woman's own health needs with her perceived responsibility for the family's health. For example, health promotion campaigns to reduce heart disease will focus on women as family health carers in advocating low cholesterol diets and exercise. Such campaigns are not usually balanced by stressing the need for good family systems (i.e. male spouses) to share responsibility for nutrition or child care so women can reduce stress, and take exercise in the interests of their own health care. Similarly, campaigns on healthy pregnancy place the emphasis on producing a healthy normal weight infant, not on the long-term consequences for women of ill health or risk behaviour while pregnant.

SOCIO-DEMOGRAPHIC FACTORS

The *National women's health policy* (1989), asserts that health providers and researchers have emphasised the significance of the lower level of status women experience in most societies. It identifies the way in which this methodological bias has been used to explain why women exhibit a higher incidence of mental health problems. The American Association of Women in Psychology at their 1988 convention drew attention to the detrimental effect of norms and practices inherent in most societies, which discriminate against and undervalue women and their activities. It pointed out how such norms are perpetuated in schools, religious institutions, the home and the workplace, undermining a woman's ability to maintain psychological and emotional well-being. Women's work, for example, is usually valued less than men's or not recognised as real work at all (e.g. their work in the home) and they have less political and economic power in society.

In the US, several studies have been conducted which identify a clear relationship between mental illness and class. Murphy (1988) reports that working class married women with young children have the highest rates of depression, while Makosky (1982) notes that sole parent women, dependent on social security and living in poor housing, also frequently suffer from depression. However, in Australia the picture is not as clear. Broom's 1984 study of class and health status found that income was a stronger indicator. For middle aged and elderly women higher rates of morbidity were associated with lower income.

Migrant women are also disproportionately more likely to be labelled as depressed. It is possible that many of these women are unlikely to understand the ramifications of the labelling process. Chiu (1983) has identified the main 'at risk' groups to be elderly and working immigrant women. She also notes that schizophrenic states are very high in eastern European females. Senile brain disorders have much higher rates in British born immigrants than in the Australian born population. She concludes that this latter finding may be artifactual, reflecting the predominance of older persons amongst British immigrants. Carmen, Russo and Miller (1981) highlight the lack of multicultural and multiracial models for understanding sex role stereotyping and sex bias on the development, diagnosis and treatment of mental disorders in women. These data add weight to the argument that social inequality is a contributor and in some cases the precursor of mental illness in women.

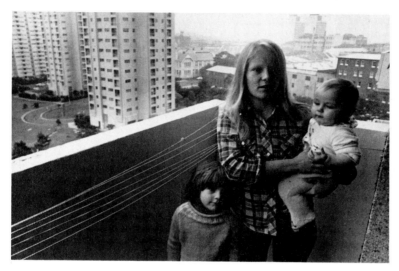

Sole parent women, dependent on social security and living in poor housing frequently suffer from depression

FEMINIST THEORIES

Feminist theory and analysis have arisen out of recognition of the realities of women's lives. Forster (1989) points out that coming to an agreement on which feminist goals shall be pursued is not easy. Many feminist theorists have chosen to see women's mental illness as wholly initiated and based in our inequitous society. They argue that we are all products of our society and, as such, have internalised many of society's expectations. Such a view does little to dispel the stigma of victim and sense of blame that mental illness invokes. It externalises all blame onto society and, by association, identifies women as passive victims.

It is not enough, however, to be merely aware of societal expectations and to have an intellectual understanding of the processes of socialisation. Feminist analysts suggest that if we ignore our internal struggles, the struggles of women will be doomed. Unconscious sources of self-defeating behaviour must be identified and addressed. Other dangers of fighting only on the societal front include: the possibility of losing women's ability to affiliate with others in bonds of affection, and often at the same time, the quest for greater self-direction. Baker-Miller (1982) suggests that women acknowledge and build on these qualities and use them as a source of strength. Relating to other women and sharing strengths and networks can, according to Furler, be an effective strategy to combat the negative influences on the mental health of women.

PRACTICAL ISSUES

Chesler (1972) commented that: female unhappiness is viewed and treated as a problem of individual pathology. Thus, a broad range of disorders, illness, sickness, disease and diagnosis are included under the umbrella of mental illness. They include:

- depression (most common);
- eating disorder (anorexia nervosa or bulimia nervosa) (see chapter eight);
- psychosomatic disorders;
- neuroses;
- situational stress response, where the focus is automatically on the response and its appropriateness;
- situational stressors, e.g. incest, rape (see chapter 11); and
- drug dependence (see chapter ten).

There are several types of therapy available at present:

- physical therapies, e.g. psychotropic drugs, electroconvulsive therapy, hormones;
- psychotherapy — individual or group;
- family therapy and community/social therapies, e.g. consciousness raising groups and hospitalisation.

According to Davis and George (1988), the *Australian health survey* identifies mental disorders as the conditions which account for the longest periods of hospitalisation for females (100.9 days).

PROVIDERS OF SERVICES

Providers of mental health care are predominantly male — especially in the more powerful areas of psychiatry and psychology (see chapter five). It is important to note the attitudes of these therapists towards women. In 1974 Fabrikant found that both male therapists and male patients agreed that women can be satisfied and fulfilled solely through the role of wife-mother. Also in 1974, the American Psychological Association found that sex role bias and sex role stereotyping were prevalent in psychotherapy. This was manifest as:

- fostering traditional sex roles;
- bias in expectations and devaluation of women;
- sexist use of psychoanalytic concepts, e.g. avoidance of the reality of incest, the maternal deprivation theory;
- the notions of mother induced schizophrenia; and
- responding to women as sex objects, including seduction of women clients.

The last issue is still the least explored. Chesler (1972) cites Masters and Johnson:

if only 25% of these specific reports (made by women about having sexual relations with their therapists) are correct, there is still an overwhelming issue confronting professionals in this field.

Saltman and Ray (1986) attest to a similar situation in Australia across the whole of the medical profession. Two opposing views have developed, both of which have implications for women undergoing psychotherapy. The traditional view is that sexual relations between therapist and patient are ethically improper. It is assumed that the therapist (usually psychiatrist, usually male) is in a powerful position in the relationship and abuses this power by coercing the female patient into sexual intercourse. This view presupposes that the woman has no power to refuse or agree. Whilst the woman patient remains victim and blameless, the male therapist is able to maintain control and power. This process often includes collusion with colleagues and denial of the event. If the event is uncovered, blame may be apportioned once again to the woman.

FEMINIST RESPONSES

Principles of therapy

Initially, the use of feminist principles in therapy placed great emphasis on the development of social and political awareness in women through the use of consciousness raising groups. These groups performed three functions:

- they helped women concentrate on looking at the condition of all women in society;
- they served to reduce the sense of isolation and alienation that many women felt; and
- they also gave women a framework for use in beginning to make sense of their own experiences.

However, it soon became apparent that, for many, understanding the social basis of women's oppression was not enough. Women sought to combine individual, group and societal processes.

Therapy groups were the natural progression. In these groups the principles and practice of consciousness raising groups were combined with some principles of psychotherapy. Individual therapy is becoming more available. Broadly, the aims of feminist therapies are to broaden the role concept for women, whilst validating and valuing what women are and do. Mander and Rush (1974) call for an end to confining and artificial sex role stereotypes. Many of the models work on increasing self-esteem, encouraging independence and responsibility for change. By helping women to recognise that they have more choices in life, they are able to strive to bring about positive change in their lives (see chapters six and eight).

However, there still remains an economic bias in access to feminist psychotherapists. Unfortunately, these services are very costly as they are neither subsidised by the National Health Insurance Scheme (Medicare), nor private health care funds. Consequently, while feminist therapy remains a solely user pays system and

Notes on Feminist Counselling

Society's Characteristics of Women

nice	less bright than men
passive	dependent
helpless	geared toward marriage
pretty	maternal
emotional	always there
caring	conforming
unstable	dependent on hormonal cycle
giving	supportive
sensitive	victims
bitchy	gossip
fickle-minded	not logical
put other's needs ahead of own	intuitive
	temperamental

Feminist Counselling

1. Woman-oriented perspective
2. Ceasing to blame women
3. Not assume equality in female/male relationships
4. Find her strengths, good feelings about herself
5. Some 'weaknesses' are strengths eg. emotional, sensitive, intuitive
6. Rediscover/re-define women's relationships with each other
7. Value other women (and self)
8. Value friendships
9. Self image (own evaluation)
10. Particular relationships reflect wider society
11. Challenge stereotypes and roles
12. Introduce new options
13. Share common concerns
14. Loving self
15. Trusting self
16. Equal relationships
17. Share professional skills
18. Reduce power difference, de mystify, contract, client as expert on herself
19. Value assumptions
20. Client's right to choose/refuse your perspective
21. Anger
22. Consciousness raising — ACTION
23. Get in touch with her wants and needs

A workshop with Sue Beecher, *Women workers in health care conference*, November 1985

the 'users' are socio-economically disadvantaged, there will be little support in an enterprise driven system for formal mental health training that has a feminist perspective. Even if the financial disincentives could be overcome, there would be little support to establish a system of training that would question the adequacy and power of the current model.

Issues of class/race and how they affect access to and appropriateness of therapy are unknown. One can only postulate that these issues are inadequately addressed (see chapter 13).

VISION FOR THE FUTURE

As with any area touched by the new scholarship on women, it is possible to chart the developmental phases through which the mental health of women has been viewed and altered. McIntosh (1984) has developed a scheme which she uses to delineate this process in relation to women's role in history. The five phases of transformation of history are applicable to the context of mental health. Rosser's paraphrasing of the scheme is included here. In brackets are the mental health equivalents:

Phase I: Womanless history. This is the very traditional approach to the discipline, which is exclusive in that only great events and men in history are deemed worthy of consideration.

Phase II: Women in history. Heroines, exceptional women or an elite few, who are seen to have been of benefit to culture as defined by the traditional standards of the discipline are included in the study.

Phase III: Women as a problem, anomaly, or absence in history. Women are studied as victims, as deprived or defective variants of men, or as protesters, with 'issues'. Women are at least viewed in a systemic context, since class, race, and gender are seen as interlocking political phenomena. Categories of historical analysis still are derived from those who had the most power.

Phase IV: Women as history. The categories for analysis shift and become racially inclusive, multifaceted, and filled with variety; they demonstrate and validate plural versions of reality. This phase takes account of the fact that since women have had half of the world's lived experience, we need to ask what that experience has been and to consider it as half of history. This causes faculty to use all kinds of evidence and source materials that academics are not in the habit of using.

Phase V: History redefined and reconstructed to include us all. Although this history will be a long time in the making, it will help students to sense that women are both part of and alien to the dominant culture and the dominant version of history. It will create more usable and inclusive constructs that validate a wider sample of life.

CASE STUDY

They were happy but exhausted. Andrew's wedding had been a great success. It was wonderful to see the family and friends together. It happened so rarely these days. As Maria and her husband drove home from the reception she could hardly believe that the next day they would be at the airport to farewell their youngest son and his bride before they travelled half way around the world to begin exciting new careers.

Maria's father had been nostalgic at the wedding reminiscing about how he and his bride had migrated from Italy to Australia half a century ago. Maria was grateful to her parents, because they had worked long and hard in their new country. Maria had not had to work while her children were growing up. She had been busy enough, though, supporting her husband

and two children. And what pride she felt when she looked at her two boys — both had graduated from university. John came home for the wedding from his job interstate, but he didn't seem to have any plans to marry soon, or work any closer to home, Maria thought.

Three months later Maria received a letter from Andrew. It was long, newsy and crammed with enthusiastic details about their new life. Rather than sharing their joy, it made her cry. In fact, she had been very tearful recently. Almost everything made her sad. In fact, that was the problem. There didn't seem to be anything to be glad about any more. She had planned to do all kinds of things when the children left home, but actually she found herself sitting around a lot and recently had been sleeping poorly, waking early in the mornings and being unable to get back to sleep. On reading Andrew's letter, she felt awful because the future seemed so bleak that she doubted she would see them again. Why did nobody understand these bleak feelings that kept overcoming her more and more of late?

Even her own mother kept saying 'What is the matter with you? You've got everything we worked so hard to give you. A nice house, a good husband, no money worries, your sons are well and happy.'

Maria answered 'I don't know who I am. Who am I, apart from somebody's wife, somebody's mother, somebody's daughter, somebody's housekeeper?' Her mother was horrified and insulted, and stormed out of the house.

A friend suggested that she should visit her general practitioner, and perhaps she could give her tablets to make her feel better. Maria thought that sounded ridiculous — she wasn't sick, was she......?

REFERENCES

Australian Bureau of Statistics (1982). *Australian health survey 1977–78: outline of concepts, methodology and procedures used*, Cat. No. 4323.

Baker-Miller, J. (1982). *Toward a new psychology of women*, Pelican, London.

Bardwick, J.M. & Douvan, E. (1971). Ambivalence: the socialisation of women, in Gornick, V. & Moran, B.K. (eds), *Women in sexist society*, New American Library, New York.

Bart, P. (1971). Depression in middle-aged women, in Gornick, V. & Moran, B. (eds) *Women in sexist society*, pp 163–186, New American Library, New York..

Broom, D. (1984). The social distribution of illness: is Australia more equal? *Social science and medicine*, 18, (11), 909–17.

Broverman, I.K., Broverman, D.M., Clarkson, F.E., Rosenkrantz, P.F. & Vogel, S.R. (1970). Sex role stereotypes and clinical judgements of mental health, *Journal of consulting and clinical psychology*, 34 (1), 1–7.

Calvert, S. (1979). Psychology and oppression, *Broadsheet*, September, No 2.

Carmen, E., Russo N.F. & Miller J.B. (1981). Inequality and women's mental health: an overview. *American journal of psychiatry*, 138, 1319–1329.

Chesler, P. (1972). *Women and madness*, Avon Books, London.

Chiu, E. (1983). Psychiatric aspects of ethnic population in Australia, *Medicine international*, 33, (1), 533–55.

Chodorow, N. (1978). *The reproduction of mothering: psychoanalysis and the sociology of gender*, University of California Press, Berkeley.

Davis, A. & George, J. (1988). *States of health: health and illness in Australia*, Harper & Row, Sydney.

Evers, H. (1985). The frail elderly woman: emergent questions in aging and women's health, in Lewin, E. & Olsen, V. (eds) *Women, health and healing: towards a new perspective*, Tavistock, London.

Forster, P. (1989). Improving the doctor patient relationship: a feminist perspective, *Journal of social policy*, 18, 337–361.

Freud, S. (1900). *The interpretation of dreams*, Standard edition of the complete psychological works, Hogarth Press, London.

Furler, E. (1985). Women and health: radical prevention, *New doctor*, 37, September, 5–8.

Janeway, E. Psychiatry and the women's movement, in *Contemporary textbook of psychiatry*, vol. 3, pp 3160–3172.

Kupinski, J. & Mackenzie, A. (1979). Study of the effects of psychiatric hospitalisation upon the well-being of the family, *Poverty and mental illness*, AGPS, Canberra.

Lee, S.H. (1979). Women and health: effects of marriage, employment and parenthood, *Community health studies*, 11, 225.

Makosky, M. (1982). Sources of stress: events or conditions, in Belle, D., *Lives in stress: women and depression*, Sage Publications, USA.

Mander, A. & Rush, A. (1974). *Feminism as therapy*, Random House, USA.

McIntosh, P. (1984). Interactive phases of curricula revision, in Rosser, S.V., *Teaching science and health from a feminist perspective*, Pergamon Press, New York.

Mitchell, J. (1975). *Psychoanalysis and feminism*, Pantheon Books, New York.

Murphy, M. (1988). Women and mental health, in Worcester, N. & Whatley, M., *Women's health: readings on social, economic and political issues*, Kendall Hunt, USA.

National women's health policy (1989). *National women's health policy: advancing women's health in Australia*, AGPS, Canberra.

Raphael, B. (1984). *Problems of mental ill health and their relevance for the Australian community*, RANZCP, Sydney.

Reynolds, I. & Rizzo, C. (1979). *Psychosocial problems of Sydney adults*, Health Commission of NSW, Sydney.

Russo, N.F. & VandenBos, G.R. (1980). Women in the mental health delivery system, in Silverman, W.H. (ed.) *A community mental health sourcebook for board and professional action*, Praeger, New York.

Saltman, D.C. & Ray, S. (1986). *Is sex really necessary: sexual innuendo in the doctor patient relationship*, University of New South Wales, Kensington.

Smith, D. & David, S. (eds) (1975). *Women look at psychiatry*, Press Gang, New York.

Thomas, K.L. (1985). Mental health objectives for women in the Australian community, *Women's health in a changing society*, Proceedings of the 2nd national conference on all aspects of women's health, Adelaide, September.

Touyz, S.W. & Beaumont, P.J.B. (1985). *Eating disorders: prevalence and treatment*, Williams and Wilkins, Sydney.

Weissman, M.M. & Kellerman, G.L. (1977). Sex differences and the epidemiology of depression, *Archives of general psychiatry*, 34, 98–111.

Women's Health Policy Committee (1985). *Women's health services in New South Wales, final report of the Women's Health Policy Committee NSW*.

10 Women and Substance Abuse

This chapter will explore substance abuse in women using psychotropic drugs as an example of dependence within the context of the health care system. Alcohol dependence will be used as an example of substance abuse, the causology of which may be unrelated to the health care system.

WHAT ARE DRUGS?

The Macquarie Dictionary (1982) defines a drug as: 'a chemical substance given with the intention of preventing or curing disease or otherwise enhancing the physical or mental welfare of men or animals; a habit-forming medicinal substance/a narcotic; any ingredient used in chemistry, pharmacy, dyeing or the like, a commodity that is overabundant, or in excess or demand in the market; etc.' In this definition there are two linked assumptions: that drugs are prescribed to enhance aspects of life and that they achieve this objective. In the case of psychotropic drugs neither of these assumptions are correct.

Psychotropic drugs refer specifically to mind altering substances, and include tranquillisers (minor and major), hypnotic/sedatives (both legal and illicit, e.g. heroin), anti-depressants and stimulants (caffeine). Broadly speaking, they can also include alcohol and nicotine.

THE FEMINISATION OF TRANQUILLISERS

Triggers to substance dependence

Sutton et al. (1986) assert that at the 1986 workshop, *Women and tranquillisers*, four major triggers involved in substance dependence were identified:

- low self esteem;
- guilt;
- shame; and
- conflict.

These triggers may be the direct result of the changing social context of women, which no longer forces them to maintain their traditional roles. Conflicts arise between the established role of mother, housewife and the newer role of paid worker. Blaze-Godsen (1987) believes that women then take psychotropic drugs in the belief that these drugs will help them cope. Mant (1986) believes that the expectations of women are so great that they adopt the 'super woman mentality' and resort to medication to maintain this role.

Other life experiences of women may contribute to triggering substance dependence. Chaiken (1986) identifies the guilt of the sexual assault victim as a trigger to substance abuse. In her report to the Women and tranquillisers conference in NSW, she asserted that 70 per cent of women with drug problems who present to agencies have had an incest or sexual assault experience.

Chaiken (1986) also highlights the plight of women in 'caring positions looking after members of the family who were sick'. She suggests that these women 'were using benzodiazepines to sleep and for their nerves'.

Collier (1987) believes that there is a connection between sexuality and drug use. He asserts that women's self esteem is in part determined by successful relationships. With paternalistic understanding, he accepts that 'drug use is an understandable option for women in this time of tension between the old and new ways of being'. In support of this theory he cites a British study that found that just under 70 per cent of women in drug treatment were dissatisfied with their sexual behaviour. Similar studies have not been conducted into the coping mechanisms of men in new style relationships. It is therefore difficult to determine whether this finding is artefactual, another form of victim blaming or a true representation.

Sargent (1984) believes that society fosters dependence in women on men, both economically and psychologically. She relates women's drug use to their position in life. Her theory is supported by studies in many countries, including Australia, Canada, Europe, Japan and New Zealand, which show that the most likely women to receive prescriptions were in the following categories:

- poor;
- uneducated;
- urban dwelling;
- housewives;
- unemployed;
- elderly;

- migrant;
- living alone.

The social practices of women also determine their substance abuse. Furler (1985) believes that 'the w../women use drugs fits in with ... what is feminine for women.' Of those people taking psychotropic drugs, there are twice as many women as men, i.e. 4–7 per cent of men compared with 7–18 per cent of women at any one time, according to the *Australian health survey* (1983). According to Cooperstock (1979) women are taking 67–72 per cent of all psychotropic drugs prescribed. She asserts that women are more likely to be prescribed tranquillisers even if they complain of the same symptoms as men.   Women are also more likely than men to receive multiple prescriptions.

The tendency has developed for women's emotions/feelings, e.g. tension, anxiety or depression to become increasingly medicalised.   These feelings can often be seen as symptoms of illness needing treatment, rather than as responses to intolerable or difficult life stresses or 'normal' variations in mood.

The role of the medical profession

Most psychotropic drugs are prescribed by general practitioners.   In particular, most benzodiazepines are prescribed by general practitioners — about 70 per cent in Australia and Canada and 65 per cent in the United States. This is despite the fact that the *General health questionnaire study* in Australia showed that 40 per cent of all adults complain of symptoms of emotional distress at any one time.

Medical consultations are a part of all women's lives (see chapter five). It has been suggested that the higher rate of prescriptions for women may be attributed to this higher number of visits to a general practitioner.

Cooperstock was the first, in 1976, to propose an explanatory model which attributes the high rate of prescriptions among women to general practitioners who adhere to a view of emotional instability in women. Her model suggests that women are permitted greater freedom than men to express their feelings, and that women perceive their feelings more readily and hence recognise emotional difficulties. This recognition enables women to define difficulties within a medical model and thus bring them to the attention of medical practitioners. Medical practitioners represent the society that sanctions this freer expression among women and therefore expect female patients to be more emotional and to require a higher proportion of mood altering drugs than the less expressive male patients.

This result could be explained in either or both of two ways:

women presenting with specifically female problems (menstrually related conditions, etc) may have the physiological bases of these trivialised and may therefore receive treatment for emotional disorders; and men and women presenting with the same symptoms of the same conditions will be treated differently.

Many overseas studies conclude that women are viewed in our society as more emotional than men. Chancellor et al (1977) also found that Australian general practitioners overestimated emotional and social problems in middle aged and elderly women and underestimated these problems in young and middle aged men.

The role of doctor as a powerful figure, particularly in the male doctor/female patient situation may accentuate the powerlessness of women and facilitate the drug answer. Melville and Johnson (1982) suggest that 'medical practitioners are trusted to exercise judgement'. They conclude that 'the image of universal healer demands that he (the doctor) must have a solution for every problem ... In practice it may mean a pill for every ill.'

In the United Kingdom, Lacey et al. (1985) surveyed 2000 people, the majority of them women, who had used tranquillisers. The process of tranquilliser prescribing was outlined in the following way:

- less than half the patients knew that they had been prescribed tranquillisers;
- less than 10 per cent were warned about side effects; and
- over 90 per cent were given repeat prescriptions of up to four months supply.

In relation to long term use;

- over 60 per cent of the patients had been taking tranquillisers for over five years;
- 40 per cent had taken them for over ten years; and
- of the respondents who had attempted to give up tranquillisers (93 per cent), 57 per cent of them succeeded.

Melville and Johnson (1982) acknowledge that such data reflect antiquated prescribing habits and they accept that there has been a recent change in the attitudes of medical practitioners.

In addition, Australian medical practitioners have often received inadequate, if any training, in psychotropic drug use. Doctors who graduated before 1960 had no formal training in benzodiazepines and those graduating after 1960 received little training. To date, they still do not receive any formal training which relates the social context of substance abuse for women with prescribing of psychotropic drugs. Lack of knowledge reinforces stereotypes. In the absence of adequate training and official drug information, health providers, particularly male, consider women patients to be by definition more neurotic, rather than realising that many of their woman patients are in situations which would make anyone neurotic. The dependence of medical practitioners on drug prescribing therefore leads them to prescribe psychotropic drugs.

Cooperstock (1979), after an extensive review of women's psychotropic drug use, has concluded that the differences in rates of visits to general practitioners by women do not wholly account for the differences in prescribing rates.

The role of the pharmaceutical industry

The pharmaceutical industry is an umbrella term for many multi-billion dollar, multi-national concerns. Approximately one third of their total sales revenue is spent on influencing the prescribing behaviours of medical practitioners. This process has been described on both sides of the Atlantic.

In the United States, Mendelsohn (1982) asserts that pharmaceutical companies sponsor direct to physician advertising (13 per cent of their total sales revenue), they provide money for medical research (9 per cent of their total sales revenue) and offer medical practitioners many other incentives to prescribe their products (e.g. free samples, promotional give-aways, computers, etc).

In Great Britain, it is estimated that pharmaceutical companies spend 20 pence of every pound of total expenditure on promotion and advertising (compared with three pence in the pound for research). The companies also send representatives to visit general practitioners. Klass (1975) has estimated that there is one drug representative for every seven general practitioners. The companies send free journals and promotion materials and advertise extensively in the journals read by doctors. It has been estimated that in Britain, on average, a general practitioner is exposed to three hundred drug company advertisements per week. Melville (1984) notes 115 advertisements in United Kingdom publications, for hypnotics and tranquillisers, of which 91 showed women as patients or had a female symbol. Only one male patient was shown.

In Australia, Wyndham (1982) has also written about pharmaceutical advertising with conclusions consistent with the overseas studies. She concludes that the advertisements reinforce the idea that men are stoic and independent and that women are complaining, dependent and irrational. She gives two examples of male and female advertising stereotypes in psychotropic drug advertisements:

> In one, all eyes are on the man as he confidently stands at the head of the board room table about to address the gathering. The caption reads 'Anxiety under control with Brand X.' In the other, a woman is shown clutching her head, with an overflowing basket of clothes and ironing board in the foreground and children playing in the distance. The caption reads 'Brand Y, when the plea is "I can't cope".'

She comments:

> The man in the advertisement is a leader/winner and the woman, a follower/loser. People are valued according to the work they do. The man is at the top of the executive ladder, the women is doing household chores for no money. The messages to doctors implicit in these two advertisements are men can control the board room, women can't even cope with the ironing board.

Mant (1986) examined 500 drug advertisements drawn from seven years of *The medical journal of Australia* and the *Australian family physician*. She found significant differences between advertisements for psychotropic and other categories of drugs and concluded that:

> The legitimacy and social impact of the patient's complaint appeared to differ for males and females. Men's illness were shown as painful interruptions of normal life and work, whereas women's ills were often shown as inconveniencing others.

There has been some controversy in Australia as to whether pharmaceutical companies are effective in self regulation of their advertising. In an independent assessment of the Australian Pharmaceutical Manufacturers' Association Code of Conduct, Moulds, Bochner and Wing (1986) found that one in three of all the advertisements in their sample of 138 could be considered misleading or containing unjustifiable claims. When these claims are combined with sexist images of the roles of men and women, it is not surprising that drug advertising is seen as not giving doctors 'balanced information in advertisements for the drug they prescribe'.

WHAT CONSTITUTES SUBSTANCE ABUSE?

Psychotropic drugs

There are four types of psychotropic drugs:

- antidepressant agents, such as amitriptyline and doxepin (commonly known as Elavil and Sinequan);
- mood normalising medications, e.g. lithium and carbamazepine, (commonly known as Lithicarb and Tegretol);
- antipsychotic medications, e.g. chlorpromazine and thioridazone (commonly known as Largactil and Mellaril); and
- antianxiety medications or benzodiazepines, e.g. diazepam and oxazepam, (commonly known Valium and Serepax).

Each of these groups have a dependence potential.

The use of chemical substances to alter feelings and behaviour is condoned and sometimes encouraged by our society, but abuse of these substances is condemned. However, social sanction makes it easy to cross the vague line between use and abuse.

Griffith-Kenney (1986) maintains that:

> substance abuse occurs when certain mood-altering substances are used inappropriately or in excess so that they alter the individual's physical and emotional integrity. Chemical dependency is a serious health problem, as well as a major social problem that affects the individual, family and community.

Many of these drugs have side-effects similar to the symptoms that they were prescribed for. The dilemma of assessing whether a particular symptom or set of symptoms is due to the drug or the original problem becoming worse is often impossible to resolve. This can result in prescribing/taking bigger doses. Many women are prescribed psychotropic drugs because they are experiencing distress resulting from distressing situations. They are being offered a medical solution to what, intrinsically, are non-medical problems. However, because the underlying problems causing the distress in the first place don't change, the woman may become further trapped in the situation because she is too 'doped' to look for alternate solutions.

Aside from the problems of tolerance/dependence/addiction and withdrawal, there can be complications, particularly if drug taking coincides with pregnancy and breastfeeding. As well, there is an increased risk and incidence of accidents (especially if combined with alcohol) and increased mortality due to overdose.

Cohen (1985) suggests that withdrawal symptoms will occur in about 40 per cent of women who have been using a benzodiazepine regularly. Ashton (1984) goes further to suggest that the development of tolerance to these drugs can mean that complete recovery may take a year or more.

The rise of the pharmaceutical industry has resulted in increased numbers and amounts available. Since the early 1960s, with the discovery of Librium and Valium, there has been an increased use of these drugs. In fact, Lader (1981) notes that in 1984–85 more than 6 million tranquilliser prescriptions were issued in Australia.

STRATEGIES FOR PREVENTION OF SUBSTANCE ABUSE

Both individual and social solutions are needed. Many non-drug solutions are available for women who feel they cannot cope with their situation. These include courses in stress management and assertiveness training, counselling, relaxation, meditation, massage, possibly herbal alternatives and acupuncture.

Providers and consumers needs to be educated about the problems associated with drug 'solutions' to non-drug problems. Women don't necessarily want a prescription just because they discuss their emotional problems.

An example of this approach is the *Women and tranquillisers community education program*. It incorporates not only the notions of the consumer's rights to ask for information from general practitioners, but also the use of emotional energy and social support in providing the consumer with the power to change the situations which are causing stress and anxiety. If women's abuse of tranquillisers and alcohol have had any positive function at all, it may be that they have drawn attention to the importance of the consumer's perceived sense of power and her access to information concerning her health.

Mant offers the following solutions to the five distinct explanations she identifies for the persistent gender bias in the use of prescription psychotropics:

- if it is true, that more women than men suffer from psychiatric disturbance, then we should be pushing for measures to improve women's health and supports;
- if it is more socially acceptable for women to go to the doctor than men, then we can encourage women to go elsewhere for help — where other treatments are offered;
- since it is more socially acceptable for women to admit to having symptoms, particularly symptoms of emotional distress, then we can try to encourage doctors to feel they do not need to treat every reported symptom — or at least not with drugs;
- whilst general practitioners are still predisposed to diagnose neurotic disturbance in women, we need to change the image of women in society — and improve the teaching about women's health for all doctors;
- since doctors are predisposed to medicate women who are experiencing psycho-social disturbance, we need to change the position of those women in society.

Much can be achieved by providers and consumers being aware of the problems faced by women and working towards social changes that generate a wider range

'This woman is now in charge' — The South Australian Women and Minor Tranquillizers Campaign

The Women and Minor Tranquillizers Campaign was conducted in three phases over a period of three years. The campaign was designed and co-ordinated by the four Women's Health Centres in South Australia, with assistance from other interested health workers in specific regions.

Aims of the campaign

The longterm goals of the campaign were directed to two main target groups: health professionals and their organizations and agencies in direct contact with the health and welfare concerns of women in the community; and women, as both users and potential users of the drugs.

With the limited resources of the campaign we recognized that we would not be able to compete with the persuasion power of drug companies in influencing prescribing patterns of the medical profession. However we aimed to develop the potential of women as active health care consumers to demand more informative and participatory health care from health services.

Philosophy

1. Women have the right to understandable information about their health care options. (For example, minor tranquillizers are addictive and ineffective as long term treatment of sleep disturbances or anxiety.)
2. With this information, women have the right to participate in decision making about their health care. (For example, whether to withdraw or not.)
3. The analysis of this problem leads to a complex web of social factors resulting in the current situation. Neither women nor doctors can be blamed or targeted as 'the problem' — the focus must be on constructive broad ranging solutions.
4. A multi-disciplinary approach to this issue is important (e.g. a range of skills and supports will be required).
5. Non-medical professionals and non-professionals have a role to play in tackling this issue. (For example, support and assistance for withdrawal can be given by any number of people given accurate information and back up.)
6. Change must occur at both an individual, community social and political level, in order to address the problem effectively.

Phase One — Research, Analysis and Resource Development

The issue was researched thoroughly by reviewing medical and sociological literature, collating Pharmaceutical Benefits Scheme and Statistics, and by a pilot survey of women attending the Menopause groups and Migrant Women's Support groups at the centre.

However, initially and most importantly, the issue was identified at the community level. A social view of health, with particular attention to the gender issues, was used in analysing the data. An action research model was adopted throughout the campaign allowing for constant review and reflection, and ongoing changes.

Phase Two — Health Worker Training

Workshops were held in four metropolitan regions and four significant country areas. This included one workshop specifically tailored to the needs of bi-cultural Italian and Greek health workers.

Strategies covered in the workshops ranged from individual counselling and support groups for withdrawal to community action and public awareness campaigns. In each region, key local workers were involved who were aware of the needs and issues in that particular community

One of the challenges not successfully met, was the active participation by doctors. Despite our zealous wish not to blame the medical profession, we suffered the full force of doctor's defensiveness. Despite our attempts to involve doctors and to acknowledge the complexity of the problems they face, we did not have the support and co-operation we had hoped for. This also reflected the 'private practice' nature of their work and their inherent difficulties in becoming involved in two day workshops and meetings. In some instances it involved their reluctance to debate the issues with other health and welfare workers who had little or no medical training. Our expectations for change in this area were far too high. A gradual and subtle input into medical training will in the end have a greater impact.

Phase Three — The Public Awareness Campaign

A Public Awareness Campaign was designed maintaining the regional focus, along with broader media coverage and debate. The campaign was launched in Rundle Mall.

Through both the launch and media releases, the issue gained considerable coverage through television, the press and radio. The display was also taken around to local shopping centres during the Public Awareness Week, where local workers were available to provide women with information and resources.

The other aspect of the campaign was a one-day 'Phone-in' giving women access to confidential information and referral. It proved to be a success, with 120 women ringing in the twelve hour period. It also attracted considerable media attention.

In retrospect a campaign focusing on sleeping problems and stress may have been less threatening to women, who were already feeling the 'collective' blame of a society that sees such issues as an individual weakness. Some women, particularly older women were slightly reluctant to approach the very public Women and Minor Tranquillizer display. It may be more appropriate in the future to have a more general women's health theme for the public display.

Adapted from 'This Woman is Now in Charge' The South Australian Women and Minor Tranquillizers Campaign, The Women's Health Centres of South Australia, paper presented to the 2nd international conference on Health Promotion, *Healthy Public Policy*, April (1988), Adelaide.

of options for women. This includes better child care, greater job opportunities, better housing.

Governments can be lobbied to provide specific venues for women to explore the issues for themselves as individuals and for women as a group e.g. women's health centres.

ALCOHOL DEPENDENCE

The National Health and Medical Research Council of Australia has recommended that the maximum intake of alcohol for women should not exceed 20 grams (one standard drink) a day. Women are more susceptible to liver damage than men. The New South Wales Drug and Alcohol Authority commissioned two studies, one in 1983 and one in 1986, into female consumption of alcohol. Both studies concluded that not only has per capita female consumption of alcohol increased dramatically in the last fifty years, but also that this reflects an increase in the percentage of women drinking, an increase in the percentage of women drinking on more than just rare occasions and an increase in the amount of alcohol consumed on each occasion.

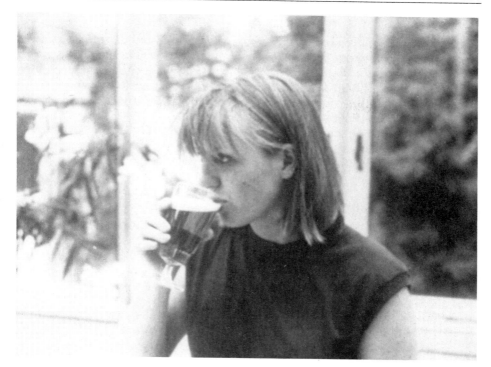

Consumption of alcohol by women has increased dramatically in the last 50 years

Sargent (1979) concludes that early researchers into women and alcohol dependence interpreted heavy drinking in women in one of two ways: either women are striving for femininity, or they unconsciously strive for masculine identification. Kinsey (1966) suggests that women alcoholics accept the traditional female role and find it gratifying. On the other hand, Parker (1975) suggests that women who exhibit alcohol dependence do so as 'a way of showing they can do what any man can do'.

Several groups are particularly at risk of developing alcohol dependence and therefore have special service needs:

- mothers, especially single mothers;
- partners of alcoholic men;
- homeless women;
- women in domestic violence situations; and
- teenage girls.

In an attempt to provide a less stereotypical view of women's drinking, Sargent (1979) undertook a study of the drinking habits of 350 female adults resident in Sydney in 1976. She found that a number of factors were associated with problem drinking:

- frequency of drinking;
- quantity of drinking;

Wine casks blamed for alcohol addiction

The ubiquitous wine cask, an Australian invention, has been blamed by a Sydney psychologist for leading more people, especially women, into becoming addicted to alcohol.

Mr Jim Maclaine, who specialises in drug and alcohol addiction at the Rosslyn Private Hospital at Arncliffe, said countless studies had proven that availability was a major contributing factor in alcohol problems.

'All the wine cask has done is to make alcohol available to people — mainly women — who would otherwise have never developed an alcohol problem,' he said.

In 15 years of therapy, Mr Maclaine said he had treated at least 1000 women who had become addicted to alcohol through casks, and he was continuing to see a sharp increase in the number of women patients.

The low price, convenience and image of respectability was making wine casks socially acceptable to women, he said.

'Without any doubt, the predominant drink of the female is wine. For as little as $6, a woman can buy a cask which has almost the same alcohol content as a case of beer — or a full litre of spirits.'

He said it was 'absurd that a dangerous, addictive and widely available chemical' was being sold for less than the price of soft drink.

The cask was deceptive because drinkers could not see the level falling.

Mr Maclaine called for the tax on wine to be increased. At present a standard four-litre cask of wine attracts a tax of only $2, while a case of beer carries a tax of $8.

'A lot of women have found it has caught up on them without any realisation of the large amounts they've been drinking,' he said. 'It can be quite subtle, starting off with the occasional couple of drinks.

'Then perhaps pressure builds up a bit, and having a drink every evening becomes a habit because it's a nice relaxant, and it helps get the cooking started.

'Reaching for the wine cask when you walk in the door is a dangerous sign that alcohol has taken a hold.'

Figures for 1988–89 from the Australian Wine and Brandy Producers' Association show that cask wine makes up 152 million litres of the total wine consumption in Australia of 312 million litres. Cask wine consumption has dropped by 7.1 per cent in the past year.

The planning and corporate affairs manager of Lindemans Wines, Mr Warwick Waddell, said there was no evidence to support claims that the advent of casks had increased alcoholism.

Paul Chamberlain, *Sydney Morning Herald*, 29 July 1989.

- never married;
- widowed;
- divorced;
- high educational level;
- location of drinking;
- drinking with friends rather than family;
- no religious affiliation;
- mother's drinking above average;
- father's drinking above average;
- husband's drinking above average.

Whilst she conceded that this information gave no indication of the cause and effect relationship, she concluded that increase in drinking accompanied increasing emancipation.

CASE STUDY

Julie knew a lot about what alcohol could do to families. Her father was a seaman. Drinking was the way he coped with the isolation of the high seas. Drinking was also the way he coped with a wife and two daughters. Maybe if he had a son it would have been different. Her mother was either out escaping her drunken husband or screaming all the time. Julie was afraid of her mother's temper. When her mother was in a bad way, she would go down to her friend Anne's place and have a cigarette.

She had started drinking in her early teens. It wasn't hard, beer was always in the refrigerator. Friday and Saturday nights were a blur, most weeks. Her circle of friends all drank a bit.

After she left school she was glad to get away from her family and she moved from her small country town to the capital city to study. The first two years at university were difficult. Most of her friends seemed distant and did not understand her behaviour. Her 'social' drinking was viewed with disdain. She didn't really know why she was doing the course anyway. It probably wouldn't lead to an exciting job, yet she didn't want to marry and have tiring, demanding children. City living was stressful and frustrating — too many queues, too many people.

Drinking helped the lonely weekends pass. But waking up with a hangover was lonely too. She knew her life was slipping out of control — that was not a good feeling. But it was so tempting to blot out these thoughts with drinking even though another part of her wanted to give up alcohol altogether.

When Jacko came along everything seemed better. He didn't look down on her drinking, in fact he drank more than she did. Did he have a drinking problem, like her father? Julie would keep him company in her room at college. They would talk, drink and smoke cigarettes. One day, when they ran out of money for cigarettes, he started shouting at her. A few weeks later he punched her about the face and ribs. Julie's friend, Anne decided it was time she stepped in...

REFERENCES

Ashton, H. (1984). Benzodiazepine withdrawal: an unfinished story, *British medical journal*, 288, 1135–1140.

Australian Bureau of Statistics (1983). *Australian health survey*, Cat. no. 4311.0, ABS, Canberra.

Blaze-Godsen, A. (1987). *Drug abuse — the truth about today's drug scene*, David and Charles, Devon.

Broverman, I.K., Broverman, D.M., Clarkson, F.E., Rosenkrantz, P.F. & Vogel, S.R. (1970). Sex role stereotypes and clinical judgements of mental health, *Journal of consulting and clinical psychology*, 34 (1), 1–7.

Carmen, E., Russo, N.F. & Miller, J.B. (1981). Inequality and women's mental health: an overview, *American journal of psychiatry*, 138 (10), 1319–1329.

Chaiken, E. (1986). Report of the NSW women and prescribed drugs working party, Women's Co-ordination Unit, Sydney.

Chancellor, A. (1977). The general practitioners' identification and management of emotional disorders, *Australian family physician*, 9 (6), 1137.

Cohen, D. (1985). *Report on phone-in for women on minor tranquillisers*, Leichhardt Women's Health Centre.

Collier, G. (1987). Benzodiazepine withdrawal, *Connexions*, 3 (7), 21.

Cooperstock, R. (1976). Psychotropic drug use amongst women, *Canadian Medical Association journal*, 115, 760–763.

Cooperstock, R. (1979). A review of women's psychotropic drug use, *Canadian journal of psychiatry*, 24 (1), 29–34.

Furler, E. (1985). Women and health: radical prevention, *New doctor*, 37, 5.

Griffith-Kenney, (1986). Substance abuse, in *Contemporary women's health*, Addison Wesley, Menlo Park.

Kinsey, B.A. (1966). *The female alcoholic: a psychological study*, Thomas, Springfield.

Klass, A. (1975). *There's gold in them thar pills — an enquiry into the medical-industrial complex*, Penguin Books, London.

Lader, M. (1981). Benzodiazepine — panacea or poison? *Australia and New Zealand journal of psychiatry*, 15, 1–9.

Mant, A. (1986). Unpublished data.

Mant, A. (1988). *Psychotropic drug use and beyond*, address to the National conference on women: alcohol and other drugs, Perth.

Melville, J. (1984). *The tranquilliser trap — and how to get out of it*, Fontana, London.

Melville, A. & Johnson, C. (1982). *Cured to death — the effects of prescription drugs*, Angus & Robertson, London.

Moulds, R.F.W, Bochner, F. & Wing, L.M.H. (1986). Drug advertising, *The medical journal of Australia*, (Letters to the Editor), 145, 178–179.

Parker, F.B. (1975). Sex role adjustment and drinking disposition of women college students, *Journal of studies on alcohol*, 36, 1570.

Report of NSW Women and Prescribed Drugs Working Party (1986). Give your feelings a better chance — try to avoid tranquillisers, Report to the NSW Premier, Women's Co-ordination Unit, Sydney.

Sargent, M. (1979). *Drinking and alcoholism in Australia*, Longman Cheshire, Melbourne.

Sargent, M. (1984). in, Haddon, C., *Women and tranquillisers*, Sheldon Press, London.

Sutton, J. (1986). *Women and tranquillisers*, Women's Co-ordination Unit, Sydney.

Wyndham, D. (1982). My doctor gives me pills to put him out of my misery, *New doctor*, 23, 21–25.

11 Women and Violence

Mateship is the most celebrated national quality, taught and glorified in schools and exploited in films in Australia. The violence inherent in the mateship ethic has never been hidden. The bushrangers, soldiers, the footballers all use violence to put down the other side. Violence performed by groups of men, or at least sanctioned by the group, is the historical heritage that provides Australian men with their mystical feelings about each other and their feelings of real power.
(Russell and Van Den Ven, 1976.)

Violence pervades this society as a method of exerting power and 'resolving' conflict. Many women have suffered and continue to suffer violence in myriad ways. Most forms of violence against women occur within the 'privacy' of the home, including domestic violence in all its guises and sexual assault, including child sexual assault. What are the implications for the health of these women? There are also many other forms of violence towards women. These include cultural mores, such as foot binding in China, clitoridectomy, and surgical mores, such as excessive rates of hysterectomy. There are also situations where violence is a work hazard and women are predominant as workers, e.g. armed holdups in banks etc., sexual harassment in the workplace.

DOMESTIC VIOLENCE

Violence is a matter of major concern for many women in Australian society. An Australia-wide survey in December 1987 found that nearly half of the population personally knows either a perpetrator or a victim of domestic violence. Violence can be described as a socially sanctioned method of exerting power and resolving conflict — it is around us all the time, on television, in the cinema, in advertising, pornography or in the form of derogatory comments.

History of domestic violence

In the late 19th century domestic violence was seen as a crime. However, by the 1920s it was seen as a problem of the individual and of his/her psychopathology. Over the next twenty years this emphasis on the individual resulted in the increasing use of psychotherapy, including relationship therapy, whereby the problem was increasingly seen as pertaining to the specific relationship. On the whole psychiatry continues to look at the problem as being one of individual psychopathology. Pizzey (1974) has written a book discussing the possibility of individual biological deficits.

By the second half of the century, shelters and refuges began in response to the needs of the women victims of domestic violence and the failure of existing agencies to assist these women. Pizzey (1974) describes in great detail the setting up of the first refuge in Chiswick in 1971. Seager and Olsen (1986) have compiled an international atlas of the development of refuges throughout the world in the first ten years of their existence. They argue that such refuges only exist by the hard work of some determined women organising locally, often with much opposition and harassment and usually without the support of local and national governments.

The refuge movement and increasing use of the law were the main instruments of the feminist response to domestic violence. The first NSW Government funded Women's Refuge opened in Sydney in 1975. Stannard (1987) reports that in 1986 over 5500 women and almost 7000 children found sanctuary in the 46 shelters operating in New South Wales. She suggests that at least 50 per cent of women seeking refuge have been physically injured and that without refuges, many of them would have been unable to find shelter and therefore returned to their homes to receive more beatings. Cox (1978) highlights that the 'beatings' may not always be physical: 'battering is not just a physical injury, it is also being told how useless you are, if you are told enough times, you start to believe it.'

The need for immediate alternative shelter is the main requirement for any woman in a violent situation. However, women's refuges provide more than mere shelter. They also provide:

- information about legal and welfare rights;
- childcare;
- professional counselling;
- support through exchange of experiences and security from further attack.

Legal definition

The New South Wales government in 1981 set up a task force to look at domestic violence. In a survey conducted by the taskforce of the major institutions which provide services for victims it was found that there was very little information to be found about the victims. None of the institutions surveyed routinely collected data. The taskforce in its report recommended that: 'hospitals, courts, including Chamber Magistrates, and the police establish and maintain adequate systems of data collection on domestic violence'.

In 1983 the *Crimes (Domestic Violence) Amendment Bill* (Section 54aa of the *Crimes Act*) came into force. Its main objective is to 'facilitate efforts to reduce the incidence of domestic violence in NSW'. Under this legislation, a 'domestic violence offence' is an assault (of any kind) committed by one person upon another where they are either married or living together in an established domestic relationship.

The role of the police force

One of the purposes of the Act was to make police take more responsibility for their actions in domestic assault cases. During their investigations, the New South Wales taskforce was quite often told of the difficulties women victims of assault face when dealing with the police. As one lawyer expressed in Stannard's article (1987):

> The police simply do not regard an assault by a husband upon his wife as a crime. They regard the assailant not as a criminal but as someone who has gone a little too far with the missus.

Victims reported to the taskforce that difficulties intensified when no visible signs of violence were evident. Hatty, a psychologist with the Australian Institute of Criminology, suggested to Stannard that the reluctance by police to act in cases of domestic assault stems from the fact that police (men) strongly identify with the husband and are thus less likely to arrest in these circumstances. Two women reported to the taskforce that they had been threatened by their husband with guns and when relating the situation to police, they were told that the police could not act until the women were actually shot. It seems the police in these cases were ignoring the *Offences Against the Person Act 1986*, which states that

> assault also ... the act of the defendant which causes to the plaintiff reasonable fear of the infliction of battery on him (sic) by the defendant. Thus a police officer laying a charge of assault does not have to rely on evidence of injury, all he (sic) needs is a reasonable suspicion that the offence has taken place.

Even the new legislation of 1983 has failed as highlighted in the 1987 *Taskforce consultation paper on violence against women and children*:

> despite the intention of the legislation, department instruction, training and increased resources, police have been slow to respond and take responsibility for cases in the way the government had hoped.

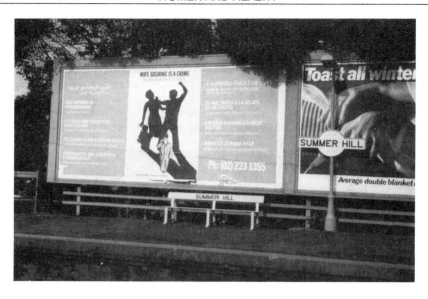

A multilingual domestic violence poster displayed on a Sydney railway station

Issues involved in family violence

> To understand family violence one must analyse the family as a social institution and the way the family unit is reproduced from one generation to the next, as well as its relationship to the wider society. (O'Donnell and Craney, 1982.)

Domestic violence is more than an individual dilemma or an occasional outburst. It is a part of life perpetuated by our beliefs, traditions and institutions. Both social customs and workforce patterns produce a structural inequality of power in relationships between men and women. Women lack economic and social powers in our present society. O'Donnell and Craney (1982) argue that the balance of family power is tipped at the outset of marriage because each partner has been constructed as a person in patriarchal society which vests power and ownership predominantly in males. This balance is tipped further when the woman is forced to become economically dependent on her husband through child-bearing. This causes her to lose her sole stake in the public world and, in many cases, her sole access to personal power.

Both within the family and the public consciousness, the assault of women within the family was shrouded in silence in Australia until the 1970s, according to Knight and Hatty (1987).

The types of domestic violence exposed in Australia include:

- severe physical violence, e.g. bruises, cuts, broken bones, burns. The O'Donnell and Saville study (1979) found that injuries ranged from severe bruising to lacerations, internal injury caused by punching and kicking, fractures, assault with a variety of weapons and attempts at strangulation

- sexual violence, e.g. rape, bondage, insertion of foreign objects
- psychological abuse, e.g. persistent verbal persecution
- financial abuse, e.g. expropriation of the wife's money
- social abuse, e.g. any of the above abuse explored outside the family context, e.g. in front of friends

Domestic violence is a part of life in many families. Women are abused within their own homes by the men with whom they have an intimate relationship. Statistics on wife battering are difficult to obtain, as incidents are under-reported and seldom identified as a separate crime. However, there is evidence through household surveys, conducted by the Australian Bureau of Statistics, to suggest that up to one third of the population may be involved.

In NSW in 1980, 11 000 women and children were given emergency shelter in women's refuges and domestic violence was frequently a factor in those cases. Many more women choose to stay.

There are many reasons why the battered woman does not leave, and pleasure from being abused is not one of them. In order to understand why women do stay, it is necessary to look at the economic, emotional and social components of the oppressed situation of women.

Griffith-Kenney (1986) postulates that women stay in abusive relationships because:

- they have negative self-concepts;
- they believe their men will reform;
- economic hardship;
- their children need their father's economic support;
- they believe divorce to be stigmatised;
- it is difficult for women with children to get work.

Another factor which makes leaving difficult is that women are brought up to believe that true fulfilment comes from being wives and mothers. This belief is often perpetuated by family and counsellors.

Knight and Hatty (1987) criticise research which suggests that unskilled women with dependent children, regardless of the socio-economic status of their husbands, are likely to be subjected to more severe and frequent levels of violence and to remain in the relationship longer than other women. They argue that quantitative data on domestic violence is misleading. It is universally agreed that wife battering knows no geographical barriers and spans all ages, income groups and nationalities.

Whilst the focus of research on domestic violence has been the victimisation of women in families, there has been a corresponding dearth of research into violent men. There is no doubt that alcohol plays a significant part in triggering violent episodes in the home, just as elsewhere. However, alcohol usage is an inadequate explanation, as it is often entirely absent. Egger and Crancher (1982), in their study of domestic violence in NSW, found that 13 per cent of their identified assailants possessed a tertiary education and 18 per cent were in professional or managerial occupations.

Needs of battered women

The needs of battered women are many. They include:

- medical treatment for injuries. Swanson (1985) suggests recognition of the battered wife may be difficult. Battered women often visit their general practitioners with complaints such as headache, insomnia, a choking sensation, hyperventilation, abdominal pain, chest pain and back pain. They may also show signs of anxiety neurosis, depression, suicidal behaviour, drug abuse and non compliance with medications.
- legal assistance
- financial assistance to provide an income for shelter, food and clothing. Means tested assistance is available from the Department of Social Security for women who leave the marital home. Some community organisations and public services offer housing assistance, e.g. the Community Tenancy Programme and the Women's Housing Co-operative.
- job training/employment counselling
- counselling to raise self-esteem and to assist them in understanding the dynamics of family violence
- an ongoing support group with counselling
- support from friends, neighbours and families. Often this support is lacking. The Royal Commission on Human Relations (1977) postulated that due to general attitudes in the community and lack of information about alternatives, many relatives encourage women to return to the marital home because their place is with their husband. This inhibition prevents women from gaining this avenue of support.

In Egger's and Crancher's (1982) study it was clear that Women's Refuges provided the most helpful service to battered women, although fewer women sought the service than say, sought that of the chamber magistrate.

INCEST

Whilst legislative definitions of incest vary, traditionally incest has always been defined as sexual contact which occurs between family members. Freud began the debate about incest and almost closed it again with his so-called 'seduction theory' (see chapter nine). Freud maintained that many of his patients' neuroses were the direct result of childhood seduction by an adult. By exposing to analytic scrutiny what was previously a taboo subject in the sexually repressive context of the 19th century, Freud explored practices that had been reported on for centuries, if only in Greek mythology. He later abandoned this theory, claiming that children fantasised about such seductions to the extent that they imagined they had really taken place. In renouncing this theory, Freud reinforced the notions of the asexual, blameless parent. Unfortunately, he introduced the concept of the lying child which until recent times has served as an excuse in following up cases of incest reported by victims.

A society at war

A loving father last week turned a gun on his three children and then on himself. It was the culmination of a fight over custody as one man struggled to continue a normal relationship with his daughter and two sons. Two adults, their solicitors and ultimately the law itself had been unable to resolve the aftermath of marital breakdown. And the result? Bloodshed.

It is now well-known that the family, apart from being the politically cherished backbone of society, is a bad place to be when things go wrong. The virtues of privacy, of self-reliance and of mutual dependence may prevent the usual protections from working when a family breaks down.

Fortunately, according to a report by Alison Wallace for the Bureau of Crime Statistics and Research, tragedies such as last week's are rare. Wallace found that in NSW, between 1968 and 1981; more than 300, or one in four, murder victims had been married to their assailants. But during the same period, only 13 children had been killed in murder-suicides. And the trend was stable.

'There are fluctuations from year to year,' Wallace said. 'But when you balance it out over a longer period, there is no discernible upward trend.'

She found that there was no real pattern in the murder-suicides that had occurred. Sometimes they came after a period of financial difficulty. But in eight out of the 13 cases, the deaths followed separation and a battle for custody of the children.

'Part of the reason is that many men find separation very difficult,' Ms Wallace said. 'The final decision to separate is often made by the woman. It follows that the women are usually under more stress up to the point of separation, but the men are more disturbed after it has occurred.'

Still, 13 dead children is 13 too many. It's a complex problem, the experts admit. After all, parents surely have the right to know their own children. But what defences do children have from the desperation of their own parents?

In NSW, the mechanism for restraining a violent man from seeing his wife and family is State law. Orders taken out under the *Domestic Violence Apprehension Act* of 1983 may offer some protection. But the Family Court which makes rulings on access to children operates in the Federal jurisdiction. Under the Australian Constitution, Federal law overrides State law whenever the two codes are in conflict. So, even if a man threatens his wife whenever he sees her, he often lawfully may continue to see his children.

Of course, a woman who believes she has a good case may go back to the Family Court and ask for the access conditions to be revised in the light of violence on the part of her former spouse. But it may be difficult, not to say expensive and time-consuming, to persuade the court that the father's rights should be overruled.

Marion Brown, a solicitor at the Women's Legal Centre in Sydney, said: 'It's a battle to get violence against spouses recognised as relevant whenever you're organising access. Violence often isn't raised in court because the solicitors advise against it. They say it's hard to provide evidence, which it often is. And they say it might look like vindictiveness on the part of the woman.'

Sometimes it is vindictiveness, says Greg Walsh, a Family Court solicitor, who doubles as the deputy chairman of the Law Society's Family Law Committee. In his practice, he has dealt with many men in a state of deep shock after marriage breakdowns. Too often, Walsh believes, difficulty in gaining access to children may push otherwise reasonable men over the edge.

'Often they're not violent before the break-up of the marriage,' he said. 'But when men have had a very close relationship with their children, it can be very difficult when their marriage breaks down. They're told they can't see their children, or they can see them only once a fortnight. They can't understand it. Sometimes they react in a violent manner.'

Walsh believes that the intervention of a third person, a counsellor, should be mandatory for any separations involving the law. At present, he points out, restraining orders may be obtained without taking any attempt to get the spouses talking.

'Just speaking to someone else in the presence of the spouse may alleviate a lot of a man's frustration,' he said. 'It's worth trying. After all, a man who's going to shoot himself and his children isn't going to worry about an order.'

Edwin Archbold, founder and co-ordinator of Families Against Unnecessary Legal Trauma, accepts Walsh's view, but believes that solicitors have to take some of the blame for custody wars.

'Solicitors have a vested interest in keeping the conflict going,' he said. 'I see people being ripped off hand over fist. You see them asking women: 'Has he been violent? Good. We can use that to stop him having access.' To me, that's a cop-out if women have put up with violence for years and years, and then they raise it in court. They should report it when it happens.'

On the front line, however, things may look decidedly different. Sue, a worker at Elsie's women's refuge in Sydney, married at 19. Sixteen years later, she is still smarting from the violence that should never have begun and should have ended when the marriage collapsed eight years ago.

'Once he bashed me because we'd run out of vegemite,' Sue said. 'But when he dragged me right across an acre block by my hair, in front of my daughter, I decided enough was enough. Even now, I hate him. We have conversations on the telephone but I still wouldn't ever be alone in a room with him.'

Her husband was eventually granted fortnightly access to their daughter. But Sue says that meant three years of being hit every second weekend when he came to pick up and drop off the child. It only ended when she left her home State and settled in Sydney. Now, the daughter sees her father in school holidays.

'I believe strongly that the men should be punished for what they're doing,' she said. 'Sure, give them counselling, but counsel them while they're in jail. No-one has the right to bash anyone. It's a crime. Of course, a reasonable man should be allowed to see his children, but if he's violent towards the woman or the children, you're doing them a favour if you keep him away. It's the community's responsibility to protect all of our children.'

Wanda Jamrozik, *Sydney Morning Herald*, July 1989.

Often in discussions concerning violence, the term 'victim' is applied. This tends to promote the notion of female passivity and may preclude individuals from taking control of life. In fact, in extreme cases, the 'victim' is held responsible for, or made to feel guilty for, the crime. Use of this term needs to be carefully analysed, as illustrated below.

For many years experts wrote quantities of non-feminist material on incest and child abuse. They blamed mothers for 'abandoning' their children to sexually deprived husbands and accused young girls of being 'seductive' or of fantasising about a sexual relationship with a male relative. Feminists have challenged these victim-blaming views: incest and child abuse occur primarily because men have power and women and children do not. They are means by which fathers, uncles and significant family contacts bolster their low self-image by taking advantage of the powerlessness of children. Men can put these motives into action because family structures allow them to misuse their power.

Incest most commonly involves fathers or stepfathers and their daughters or stepdaughters. However, other relatives and siblings may be involved. *The Incest Survey* conducted in Brisbane (1980–82) by Women's House and the *Child Sexual Abuse Report* conducted in Adelaide (1983) by the Adelaide Rape Crisis Centre suggest that the perpetrator is usually a supposedly trusted adult male and the prevalence of incest is approximately one in every five children in Australia. Brookman (1983) identifies several factors which can suggest incest:

- reversal of family roles, i.e. adolescent daughter acting as mother;
- running away;
- serious rebellion against the mother;
- low self esteem;
- parental alcoholism ;
- sexually transmitted disease or pregnancy in the incest victim.

Incest may take many forms including using suggestive language, kissing, voyeurism, petting, intercourse, oral sex and masturbation. The activity is often foreign and frightening to the child. However, the power to resist incest does not rest with the child who must constantly seek parental approval. Often these children have a history of long term abuse. Relationships with parents and near family become unsafe. Herman (1981) suggests that the effects of this abuse are life long. Difficulties with sexually intimate relationships are common as is self-blaming. Incest survivors may turn to at-risk behaviours, e.g. drugs and alcohol, to override their lack of personal safety.

SEXUAL ASSAULT AND RAPE

Hanmer and Saunders (1984) suggest that many women live in constant fear of rape and sexual violence. They assert that these women restrict their activities to daylight hours or when accompanied by a man. Brownmiller (1975) goes one step further to suggest that all women's lives are in some way restricted by this fear.

Historically, the victim was, at worst, seen as a careless woman, who had a tendency to stray. At best, women were conditioned from birth to be passive and in need of protection. In this way, the victims were at a disadvantage from the outset. Because they had no knowledge of their own power or physical strength they believed that they required a man to protect them.

As with other data which relate to women and violence, the data on women and sexual assault/rape are difficult to interpret. In 1985 the Australian Bureau of Statistics published the results of a survey which suggested that the number of sexual assaults thought to occur was four times the reported number. In 1985 Bonney tabulated statistics on sexual assault in NSW. She found that 92.5 per cent of the victims of sexual assault between 1981 and 1983 were women. The majority of these women were in the 18–25 years age group. The Health Commission of NSW, in its Survey of help centres for victims of sexual assault found that nearly 88 per cent of sexual assault victims presenting between 1978 and 1981 were of Australian, British, New Zealand or American origins. They concluded that they had difficulty obtaining data from women from aboriginal and non-English speaking backgrounds, which they attributed to the women having problems in reporting sexual assault.

In relation to social class, Bonney (1981) suggests that the social class of the victim is closely related to that of the attacker. Students, unemployed women, office workers and housewives figure highly as victims. Bush (1977) suggests that there are few cases of reported rapes of professional women in Victoria. Several conclusions are possible. Professional women have access to a wide variety of services to help them after an attack. They are more likely to be aware of the poor success rate in achieving a satisfactory end result through reporting. It may be that professional women are more likely to be assaulted by men from more professional backgrounds and therefore both groups collude to minimise reporting. Or even the possibility that professional women are more likely to associate with professional men and these men have other avenues in which they can assert their power.

Certain myths about sexual assault were dispelled by both Bonney and Bush. Over 30 per cent of sexual assaults take place in the victim's own home, thereby dispelling the myth that rape is always perpetrated by strangers and takes place outdoors. Sexual offenders are in the main psychologically normal males, supporting the feminist assertion that rape is an issue of power, not mental health. Violence does not always accompany rape. Bonney asserts that 44 per cent of all victims have no physical injuries at all and in less than 30 per cent of cases, the rapes were accompanied by the threat of weapons.

The categorisation of rape

There have been many attempts at categorising the individual who rapes, the type of rape and the sequela of rape in an effort to make a horrific act understandable. Freud viewed rape as an instinctual expression of male aggression, usually blocked by civilisation. Groth and Burgess (1977) found that one third of all rapists serving prison terms had been sexually abused as children. Repeated phone-ins conducted by rape crisis centres in Australia have found that the incidence of unreported rape is high and in such cases the perpetrator is often known to the victim.

Rapes have also been characterised according to the style and suspected motivation. Griffith Kenney (1986) identifies five categories:

- the blitz rape in which the victim and assailant are strangers and the assault occurs suddenly;
- the confidence rape in which the assailant coerces the victim into a sexual act. In a university study in the United States, Koss and Oros (1982) discovered that over 9 per cent of the male students they interviewed had attempted or committed rape in this manner without being reported;
- the power rape in which the assailant plans the rape in order to prove that he is desirable, potent and strong, involving victims both known and unknown to the assailant;
- the anger rape which often cannot be differentiated from the power rape in which the rape becomes symbolic of power and revenge. Foley and Davies (1983) suggest that this type of rape usually involves violence; and,
- the sadistic rape in which the perpetrator is psychiatrically disturbed.

The victims' response to rape has also been quantified. The sequela of rape have been medicalised into a constellation of symptoms which have been identified as the Rape Trauma Syndrome. The acute phase includes an immediate impact reaction, physical reactions and an emotional reaction to a life threatening situation. There is an immediate impact reaction. Burgess and Holstrom (1974) describe the victim as being tense during interview, crying or sobbing in describing specific acts and smiling in an anxious manner when certain issues were stated. Physical symptoms are also present. Areas of assailants' force often include the throat, chest, arms and legs. Most victims have described a general feeling of soreness all over their bodies. Specific symptoms related to the area of the body which was the focus of the attack have also been reported. Sleep and eating pattern disturbances are also common. Emotional reactions include fear, guilt, self blame, anger and revenge. After an acute phase, the victim may take some time to return to a life routine. The long-term process includes changes in lifestyle, dreams and nightmares, and phobic reactions. Crisis counselling is effective with victims developing Rape Trauma Syndrome. Additional help may also be required in the longer term.

The police

In 1983 the Police Sexual Assault Unit was set up in New South Wales. Courses in sexual assault are incorporated into police training and available to all police officers. A trained police woman is required to be available to take the statement of any sexual assault victim. In 1988 the NSW Sexual Assault Committee found that 90 per cent of legally documented sexual assaults occurring in that state were first reported to the police.

Sexual assault centres

The first of these centres was established by the Commonwealth Department of Health in 1978. Whilst governmental guidelines require that police refer all persons with documented sexual assaults to sexual assault centres, the New South Wales Sexual Assault Committee (1988) found that in 1982 less than 50 per cent of these women actually made contact with a centre.

These centres, which operate 24 hours a day, provide: medical services to deal with the physical effects as well as to collect forensic evidence, counsellors to offer support to the victim, as well as to family and friends, and community programs.

The legislation

The sections of the Crimes Act of 1900 (and Amendments of 1955) relating to rape and attempted rape were repealed and replaced by the Crimes (Sexual Assault) Amendment Act of 1981. Changes included:

- replacing the old charges of rape and attempted rape with a range of sexual offences, which included penetration of other orifices and the use of other bodily parts and foreign objects;
- incorporating the level of violence and harm into the law;
- identifying rape within marriage as a crime;
- revising penalties;
- removing the sexual reputation of the victim from admissible evidence.

In reviewing the effects of this legislation, the NSW Sexual Assault Committee released a report in 1988 highlighting key areas for further action:

- expansion of Sexual Assault Services to rural communities

- further training for police;
- simplification of court procedures;
- attending to the needs of special groups of women, e.g. aboriginal, non-English speaking background and disabled women;
- review of the necessity of committal proceedings;
- education of the legal profession to prevent cross-examination of victim on previous sexual experience and reputation;
- review of conviction rates, which have not increased significantly since the change in legislation.

Whilst the Committee identified key strategies for improving the legal implications of sexual assault for the victim, other strategies are necessary, including regular review of compensation payable under the Criminal Injuries Compensation Scheme, long term rehabilitation of sexual assault victims, review of the success of legal punishment as a deterrent, and finally, community education about rape and sexual abuse and re-education about the role of women in our society.

SEXUAL HARASSMENT

Mackinnon (1979) asserts that in terms of the work place, sexual harassment occurs when a person in a position of control uses their position of authority to coerce the other person (usually a woman) into sexual acts or relations or

Labourer 'friend' on sex attack charges

A labourer, 41, smashed the face of a woman into a car bonnet before having sexual intercourse with her at Kings Cross, police claimed in Central Court yesterday.

Police alleged the labourer later dragged the woman into a nearby Rushcutters Bay park where he hurled her over a fence and had intercourse with her.

The man, whose name was suppressed by Mr Joe La Cava, JP, appeared on two counts of maliciously inflicting actual bodily harm on the woman with intent to have sexual intercourse with her at Kings Cross early yesterday.

He was also charged with taking her by force with intent to carnally know her on Friday.

The Police Prosecutor, Seargent Jay Corr, claimed that late on Friday the man went with the woman, 'a mutual friend', to Kings Cross where he attempted to kiss her in a lane.

'She refused (his kiss) and he threw her on to the bonnet of a car and started biting her face and nose,' Sgt Corr alleged.

'He tried to have intercourse with her and grabbed her by the hair and smashed her face to the bonnet.'

A passing car disturbed the man and he dragged the woman to Rushcutters Bay.

'He told her to shut up or she would be killed,' Sgt Corr claimed.

'He tried to kiss her, then bit her face again before having sexual intercourse with her.'

Asking that bail be refused, Sgt Corr claimed the woman feared for her life if the man were freed.

Public solicitor Ms Forbes asked that the man's name be suppressed and said that he denied the charges.

Mr La Cava refused bail and remanded the labourer in custody to Central Court tomorrow.

Steve Warnock, *Sun-Herald*, 13 May 1990

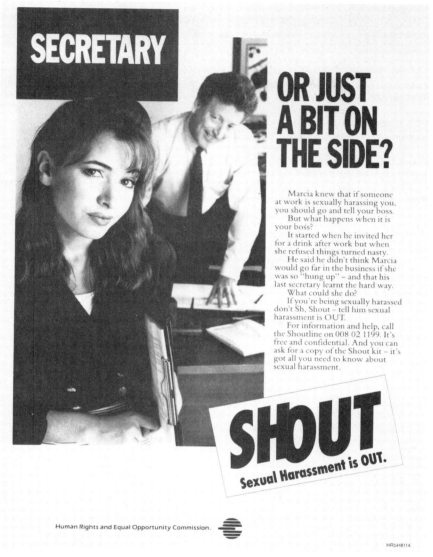

SECRETARY

OR JUST A BIT ON THE SIDE?

Marcia knew that if someone at work is sexually harassing you, you should go and tell your boss.

But what happens when it is your boss?

It started when he invited her for a drink after work but when she refused things turned nasty.

He said he didn't think Marcia would go far in the business if she was so "hung up" – and that his last secretary learnt the hard way.

What could she do?

If you're being sexually harassed don't Sh, Shout – tell him sexual harassment is OUT.

For information and help, call the Shoutline on 008 02 1199. It's free and confidential. And you can ask for a copy of the Shout kit – it's got all you need to know about sexual harassment.

SHOUT
Sexual Harassment is OUT.

Human Rights and Equal Opportunity Commission.

HRSH8114

A Human Rights and Equal Opportunity Commission Sexual Harrasment campaign, aimed at young women

punishes the person if they refuse to comply. Harassment encompasses a wide range of behaviours, from the blatantly physical e.g. rape, assault or fondling, to the more subtle, e.g. the unjustifiable downgrading of job responsibility.

In her work on sexual harassment or, as she calls it, 'women's hidden occupational hazard', Mackinnon (1979) identifies six forms of sexual harassment:

- constant ogling and leering at the female body;
- constantly brushing against the female body;

- forcing a woman to submit to squeezing or pinching;
- catching a woman alone for forced sexual intimacy;
- outright sexual propositioning, often backed by the threat of losing a job or promotion;
- forced sexual relations.

Sexual harassment is not only hidden by men, but also by the popular myths that contradict women's actual experiences. The most common myths are:

- women enjoy it;
- it is trivial and unimportant;
- it only happens to women in low status jobs;
- it is easy for women to handle.

Underlying these myths is the assumption that sexual attention to women is always flattering. Hanmer and Saunders (1984), in their community study on violence towards women, suggest that sexual harassment may have concrete negative effects on victims. They found that 75 per cent of respondents who had experienced sexual harassment and ignored it experienced intensified sexual harassment. Moreover, 25 per cent of the women who had been harassed were penalised by reprimands or sabotage of their work. Of the 18 per cent of harassed women who were strong enough to complain through established channels, more than half reported that no action resulted. It is clear that women are caught in this double bind.

Sexual harassment can also have less concrete effects as was evidenced by the Hanmer and Saunders (1984) survey. Amongst the women who did not formally complain about sexual harassment, 52 per cent thought nothing would have been done if they had complained, 43 per cent felt their complaints would have been treated lightly or ridiculed and 30 per cent felt that they would have been blamed or would have suffered repercussions. MacKinnon (1979) reported similar findings in her study. She concluded that women neither wanted to be harassed at work nor found it flattering.

CASE STUDY

Dr Penny Humphries was used to getting phone calls at three o'clock in the morning. But she was always uneasy arriving in the Emergency Department to see a woman or child who had been sexually assaulted.

This morning when she arrived in the small room the young woman huddled quietly on the narrow bed looked so hopeless. One eye was swollen and blue and when she opened her eyes they were scared and tearful. She mumbled that her name was Bernadette. Penny sat down close to Bernadette and began to talk quietly to her. With gentle prompting, Bernadette described her hours of trauma.

At five o'clock the previous afternoon she had been walking toward the railway station carrying the shopping she had bought at the local shopping centre. She was looking in the window of the jewellery shop when she became aware of two men in their early twenties laughing and joking behind her. One of them said to her 'We're taking you for a drink, sweetheart.' She refused to go and continued to walk toward the station, but they persisted in following her. Somehow she was in a car. Five hours later they dropped her back in the same place, after she had been raped by them and two other of their friends. She had lost count of the number of times they had raped her. Going round and round in her mind were indelible impressions of jeering laughter, the smell of alcohol, careless hands touching and slapping her, pain and fear, and then more pain and more fear.

During the next few hours Penny learned about Bernadette's background, undertook a complete physical examination, and helped her deal with the immediate shock of her experience. Because she was nineteen years old, and had recently moved to the town to work, Bernadette was away from her family and friends — in fact she knew almost no-one in the town.

By mid morning Penny felt that Bernadette trusted her, but that she was in no state to return on her own to her flat, in spite of the fact that she had no physical injuries that necessitated her staying in hospital. June, the unit social worker, called the co-ordinator of the local women's refuge and arranged for Bernadette to spend the next few days there.

The refuge provided a caring environment for 24 hours a day, and Bernadette looked much calmer when Penny saw her the following morning. Penny talked through the aspects of her management with Bernadette. There were three aspects. The refuge would provide support and an opportunity for her to talk through her experience. Penny herself, because of her experience in psychiatry and women's health, would provide counselling and would also discuss with her any likelihood of pregnancy. One of the things particularly worrying Bernadette was that she was in the mid-point of her menstrual cycle and could be pregnant. If so, her strong Catholic upbringing would make it very difficult for her to seek an abortion.

During the next few weeks, Bernadette's wounds, both psychological and physical, began to heal with the caring patience of all involved. However, four weeks later, when it was confirmed that she was, in fact, pregnant it was a devastating blow. Bernadette felt sick with worry one minute, and then blindingly angry the next. There were so many people involved: the police; the hospital staff; the refuge staff; the nuns at the local convent from whom she had sought advice. Powerlessness, anger and despair captured her mind, and seemed to make it impossible for her to come to a decision about anything. The fact of her pregnancy was an all consuming ethical conflict, which seemed impossible to resolve.

Looking back later she remembered the hours of discussions, counselling, crying, arguing, and silence that enabled her in the end to come to a decision about her future. More importantly, it was a decision that she felt at peace with.......

REFERENCES

Adelaide Rape Crisis Centre (1983). *Child sexual abuse report*, Adelaide Rape Crisis Centre, Adelaide.

Bonney, R. (1985). *Bureau of crime statistics and research crimes, (Sexual Assault) Amendment Act 1981 final report*, Attorney General's Department: Sydney.

Boston Women's Health Book Collective (1985). *The new our bodies/ourselves*, Penguin Books, Melbourne.

Brookman, R.R. (1983). Adolescent sexuality and related health problems, in Hoffman, A. (ed.), *Adolescent medicine*, Addison-Wesley, Menlo Park.

Brownmiller, S. (1975). *Against our will: men, women and rape*, Simon and Schuster, New York.

Burgess, A. & Holstrom, L. (1974). *Rape: victims of crisis*, Prentice Hall, Maryland.

Bush, J.P. (1977). *Rape in Australia*, Sun Books, Melbourne.

Cox, S. (1978). The better they be, *Australian social welfare*, July, 10.

Egger, S.J. & Crancher, J. (1982). Wife battering: analysis of the victim's point of view, *Australian family physician*, 11 (11), 830–832.

Foley, T.S. & Davies, M.A.(1983). *Rape: nursing care of victims*, Mosby, St. Louis.

Griffith-Kenney, J. (1986). *Contemporary women's health*, Addison-Wesley, Menlo Park.

Groth, A.N. & Burgess, A.W. (1977). Sexual dysfunction during rape, *New England journal of medicine*, 297, 764–766.

Hanmer, J. & Saunders, . . (1984). *Well-founded fear: a community study of violence to women*, Hutchinson, London.

Herman, J.L. (1981). *Father-daughter incest*, Harvard University Press, Cambridge MA.

Knight, R.A. & Hatty, S.E. (1987). Theoretical and methodological perspectives on domestic violence: implications for social action, *Australian journal of social issues*, 22 (2), 452–464.

Koss, M.P. & Oros, C.J. (1982). The sexual experience survey: an empirical instrument for investigating sexual aggression and victimisation, *Journal of consulting and clinical psychology*, 50, 455–457.

Mackinnon, C.A. (1979). *Sexual harassment of working women: a case of sexual discrimination*, Yale University Press, New Haven.

National Women's Health Policy (1989). *National women's health policy: advancing women's health in Australia*, AGPS, Canberra.

O'Donnell, C. & Craney, J. (1982). *Family violence in Australia*, Longman Chesire, Australia.

O'Donnell, C. & Saville, H. (1979). *Domestic violence and power*, Longman Chesire, Australia.

Pizzey, E. (1974). *Scream quietly — or the neighbours will hear*. Penguin Books, London.

Report of the NSW Task Force on Domestic Violence (1981). Premier's Department, New South Wales.

Royal Commission on Human Relations (1977). *Final Report*, Part 4, AGPS, Canberra.

Russell, D.E.H. & Van den Ven, N. (eds) (1976). *Crimes against women — proceedings of the International Tribunal*, Les Femmes, California.

Seager, J. & Olsen A. (1986). *Women in the world: an international atlas*, Pan Books, London.

Stannard, B. (1987). Domestic violence: the problem we don't talk about, *The Bulletin*, August 11 1987.

Swanson, R.W. (1985). Recognising the battered wife, *Canadian family physician*, 31, 823–825.

Taskforce consultation paper on violence against women and children (1987). Premier's Department, New South Wales.

Women's House (1980–82). *The incest survey*, Women's House, Brisbane.

12 Women and Occupational Health and Safety

The occupational health and safety of women in the paid workforce has only recently become an area of concern for both women workers and employers. Recently attention has been paid to several health-related issues, which are to be discussed in this chapter including occupational overuse, maternity leave, child care and superannuation. Many occupational health issues cross the boundaries between paid and unpaid work. In many areas affecting women's health at work legislation is lagging.

PAID/UNPAID WORK

The number of women in the paid workforce is steadily increasing — a direct result of the changing role of women. Not only are there social imperatives that direct women's work, but also economic necessity and a change in the reproductive window in which the span of child-rearing years has been compressed.

The duality of roles for most women as primary unpaid worker at home and paid worker may force many women to consider their employment priorities. Low status, low pay employment may provide the only avenue for women who must move in and out of the workforce during their child-bearing years. The paid/unpaid agenda of employment may have increased the complexity of occupational health issues. For example, home injury, such as domestic violence and work injury may aggravate each other.

The spectrum of work related injury in Australian women is difficult to assess. There are two separate issues:

- the case where the work is no more harmful to women than men, but the workforce is predominantly female, e.g. the beauty industry; and
- the industries where significant occupational hazards are present for women, e.g. the airline industry.

Specific hazards

Specific hazards as they affect women may relate to:

- the type of industry;
- the environment in which the women work; and
- the working conditions in that environment.

These hazards may be biological, chemical or physical. The major biological hazards are bacteria, viruses, yeasts and moulds transmitted in the work setting to hospital and health care workers, hairdressers and beauticians, laundry and dry-cleaning workers, and household workers.

Chemical hazards include cleaning liquids, hairsprays, dyes, solvents, pesticides and anaesthetic agents. Such agents particularly affect hospital workers, clerical workers, laundry and dry cleaning workers, and textile and clothing workers.

The major physical hazard is noise. Current legislation requires that noise levels in the workplace need to be below 90 decibels. At that level at least 11 per cent of exposed women will suffer hearing loss by retirement age. Another physical hazard is radiation. This is particularly important for dental technicians and hospital and laboratory workers. Women who work in the textile and clothing industry may be exposed to dust, fumes, excess heat and humidity.

Whilst these serious hazards have the potential to affect the majority of women in the workforce with life threatening sequela, the occupational health and safety emphasis has not been on the women, but rather their unborn foetuses. Mathews (1985) states that

> women are barred from employment in certain occupations, either through award provisions or through legislation, where it is considered that the work is sufficiently dangerous to interfere with the health, not of the women, but of the foetus she may carry. An example of such a prohibition is the *Lead Workers Regulations* found in many states of Australia.

Many agents that are likely to affect the foetus adversely, that is they are embryotoxic, are well known. These agents and occupations where exposure may occur include:

- lead (battery works, pigments);

- cadmium (batteries, smelters);
- mercury (felting, chlorine, electrolytic plants);
- benzene (use of solvents, glues);
- ethylene dibromide (fumigation workers);
- polychlorinated biphenyls (electrical workers, microscopists);
- carbon monoxide (brewery workers, petrol station and car park attendants);
- anaesthetic gases (operating theatre staff);
- chlordecone [kepone] (agricultural workers);
- x-rays (radiographers);
- ethyl oxide (hospital workers);
- oxfendazole [Synanthic] (veterinary and farm workers);
- ethylene thiourea (laboratory workers); and
- glycol ethers (workers who use solvents, antifreeze).

The traditional response by large companies to the problem of embryotoxic agents has been to restrict the employment of fertile women in these industries. Such a policy has had disastrous effects on the employability of women:

- it restricts their employment opportunities;
- removes responsibility from the employer to provide a workplace that is a safe and healthy place for all;
- places the onus on the woman to protect herself and future child; and
- fails to take account of the fact that many fetotoxic agents are also toxic to the male reproductive system, or are genetically toxic.

In Australia, the ACTU has not recorded such policies nor these sequela.

The work environment

The location of work environments often conforms to the needs of the industry, for instance, inaccessible locations owing to cheap rental. Industrial complexes are frequently removed from shopping areas and child care centres to prevent day time distractions, making the dual tasks of women as paid workers and unpaid domestic workers difficult.

Many work environments have been designed by men for men. Women involved in the manual handling industry often complain that workbench height, trolley size and the bulk packaging of detergents and food items are inappropriate for the majority of women workers.

Many work environments were not intially designed to be places of work. In 1984 it was estimated by the Women's Bureau of the Department of Employment, Education and Training that between 30 000 and 60 000 individuals, the majority of whom were women, were working as outworkers in their own homes. The predominant industries were clothing, process and textile work. This situation arose because in many cases these women were migrants and knew little English and outwork in these industries required no verbal or written communication skills. More recently another group of women have joined the ranks of outworkers: data entry processors. In this type of work English literacy skills are necessary. The women working in this area are often young mothers forced to do so by inadequate, expensive, inaccessible or even unavailable child care facilities either at work or in their local communities. Outworkers are the most powerless working women in the community. They have no rights concerning illness, working conditions, holiday provisions or superannuation. They are located in their own homes and therefore have little communication with other outworkers in order to form networks to change their work practices. The *National women's health policy* suggests that they are also more vulnerable to intimidation and sexual harassment.

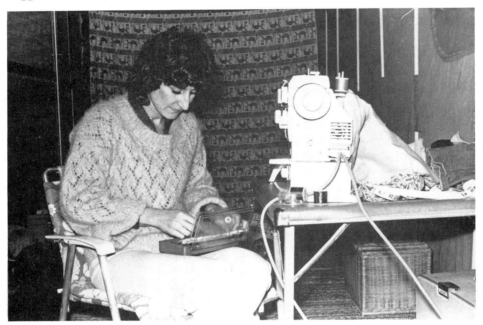

A woman outworker

The working conditions

The timing of work can have profound effects on the reproductive cycle of women. Shiftwork and erratic hours are particularly problematic for women in health care, women flight stewards, women assembly workers and women word processors.

The nature of work for some women has continued to be a controversial issue. The effects of occupational ill health on women workers are either not recognised or trivialised. For example women performing repetitive, monotonous work on key boards, are less likely to have the freedom to alter their work practices than their male counterparts. It is therefore not surprising that 62 per cent of claims made because of overuse syndrome/repetitive strain injury came from women workers.

Physical activities causing back injuries whilst well documented are poorly managed (NSW Anti-discrimination Board 1984). Weight lifting and carrying are major issues for nurses. A 1986 study by the Queensland Nurses Union of

Employees of nurses in the state of Queensland showed that nearly 50 per cent of all work-related injuries for nurses were back injuries compared with 23 per cent in the workforce as a whole. The imposition of weight restrictions as practised in other predominantly male industries has proved unworkable. The case of back injuries in nurses highlights the difficulties women in the workplace face not only identifying their legitimate occupational concerns, but also in achieving effective change in the workplace. In other industries, imposing weight lifting limits can serve to reinforce differential treatment of male and female workers. Refshauge (1986) argues that weight limits can act as a screen for prejudicial employment practices and attitudes.

Compensation

Women in the workforce are less likely to seek compensation than their male counterparts. They are also less likely to know their rights and to belong to a trade union. Seeking compensation may be so stressful for women that they choose to leave the workforce before the injury is compounded by the social, physical and mental deterioration that accompanies injury and the battle for compensation. In the private sector, women seeking compensation may have to take private legal action which places them in an adversarial position with their employers (National Women's Health Policy 1989).

The National Women's Advisory Council (1983) suggested that the low number of compensation claims made by women reflected their fear of losing their jobs. In the proceedings of their 1981 seminar, several alternative strategies to claiming compensation were raised: sick leave, holidays, or unpaid leave.

Prevention and the workplace

In the United Kingdom, the General Municipal Boilermakers and Allied Trade Union advised its regional officials in 1981 and 1984 to negotiate agreements with their employers covering:

- screening facilities on sight arranged through the women's National Cancer Control Campaign;
- paid time off for screening and follow up treatment; and
- an educational campaign for the members.

In Australia no such initiatives have been canvassed. The ACTU does not have a policy on cancer screening tests for women.

The Women's Health and Industry Project in the state of New South Wales, Australia, undertook to visit several factories in the suburb of Lidcombe. They provided women with information on health issues relevant to women, and in particular, information on cancer. They found that most women had little information regarding breast and cervical cancer screening. Even the larger factories, which have their own nurses, do not utilise these nurses to provide information on women's health issues. Most of the women in these factories work very long hours, with little time between their responsibilities of housework, child care and work to undergo cancer screening tests.

MATERNITY LEAVE

Society has extolled the virtues of motherhood while, quite incongruously, for the most part choosing not to involve itself in defraying any of the costs of maternity, on the basis that for the most part reproduction is a private issue. Communities have been at pains to reap the benefits of a growing population but have been recalcitrant in bearing any of the costs. The net effect has been to place women in the home and to view their excursions into the workplace as at most temporary and at worst a shirking of their uncompensated societal 'duty'.

Historically, the issue of maternity leave goes back as far as 1919 when the International Labour Organisation issued a convention recommending paid maternity leave for 12 weeks. The ILO extended this legislation in 1952, however, Australia did not ratify this convention. It was not until 1966 that the Liberal-Country Party coalition government introduced maternity leave without pay into the public service. This provision did not provide any job security and made it difficult for women to maintain their seniority within the service. In 1972 the Labor government amended this policy to 12 weeks paid leave and the guarantee of re-employment after confinement. By the end of the 1970s a variety of public and private awards covered 42.4 per cent of working women, many still without adequate job protection.

In more recent times the view of maternity and working women has altered quite dramatically, given that maternity leave legislation exists and is enforced and reinforced by women taking this leave as part of their rights as workers. Maternity leave has become one of the many issues involved in the struggle to improve the access of women to equal job opportunities. It has also become an increasingly important union issue particularly in the case of teachers and nurses.

The significance of the case for maternity leave in Australia can be gauged by adoption of the working women's charter by the Australian Council of Trade Unions in 1977. Maternity leave, equal pay and childcare were the priorities to be addressed by a committee set up by the ACTU in 1978.

The test case argued by the ACTU in 1978–1979 formed the basis of federal and NSW maternity leave awards. Women who are commonwealth employees are covered by the *Maternity Leave (Commonwealth Employees) Act 1973*. This provides for a maximum of 52 weeks of leave without pay. It includes accrued recreation and long service leave and the right to return to the same job. Hence the leave essentially suspends employment, while preserving continuity of service. Emphasis should be placed on the fact that maternity leave is inclusive of other leaves. That is, if one had, for example, 40 weeks of long service leave, then only 12 weeks of actual maternity leave could be taken. The person who may be employed to replace a woman on maternity leave is employed on a temporary basis only in that particular position.

In developing countries the situation is far worse, given that the health needs of pregnant women are the primary concern. Work needs come later. However, this does not mean that organisations such as WHO ignore the issue. In fact, along with the ILO, WHO supports maternity leave.

The crucial role that governments can play in providing social support to women is undeniable, but is not in itself sufficient. The main reason is that most women in developing countries are engaged in informal income-earning activities and are therefore not usually covered by the minimal social security laws (e.g. in one country in the South-East Asia Region it was estimated that protective maternity legislation covered only 1.6 per cent of the women). But even in some developed countries the underlying assumption is that difficulties arising from the combination of motherhood and employment (formal and informal) are to be borne solely by the individual (Sivard 1984).

CHILD CARE

Child care is seen by Australian women as the single biggest barrier to work. Repeated surveys have shown that this is regarded by women in the work force as having equal importance to wages. Particular problems cited were:

- finding regular child care;

Creche plans hit red tape

Anne O'Sullivan could write an episode for TV's *Yes Minister* after her experiences trying to set up a creche in Sydney.

There are 100,000 children seeking child-care places in Australia but the red tape is enough to discourage anyone from opening a centre.

A spokesperson for the Department of Family and Community Services said new legislation to be tabled in Parliament next month would update laws in force since 1939, making it easier for qualified people to operate creches.

But the move comes too late for Ms O'Sullivan. A Sydney midwife, she was pregnant when she and another nurse took plans for a creche to the then Department of Youth and Community Services.

'We told them we were interested in looking after new born to one-year-olds but the authorities said we would have to look after two-year-olds also,' she said.

Ms O'Sullivan told the department she wanted to rent premises for the creche and was given a 20-page list of regulations which included providing the department with five plans of the house.

Rules included providing outdoor space for a sandpit, using only a house facing north to north-east so it would get the morning sun, and hiring staff to do jobs they could do themselves.

Even if she had managed to get a house which complied with all regulations, she would have had to wait for approval from the department, the Board of Fire Commissioners and the local council.

Ms O'Sullivan was told it would not be a good idea for her to look after her own children at the same time as she would probably favour her child over the others, a suggestion she — a trained midwife — was insulted by.

Alternatively, she was told by the department she could set up a creche in her own home and would be allowed to take care of up to five children that way. But after adding up the costs, she realised she would only make about $200 for a 40-hour week — and gave up.

A Family and Community Services department spokesman agreed the process was frustrating.

'There is too much emphasis on physical standards like whether there are enough toilets but not enough on the quality of care, something the department wants to change,' she said.

Amruta Slee, *Sun-Herald*, 23 July 1989.

- coping with changes of the established routine, e.g. school holidays, childhood sickness; and
- lack of spouse support.

The ACTU adopted the Working Women's Charter and has appointed an occupational child care officer.

The location of child care facilities is also an important concern for working women who are mothers. Child care can be employment based or neighbourhood based.

Employment based child care

Employment based child care offers many advantages to the employer. Employers do not have be to financially disadvantaged by providing their own workplace child centres, even if they charge significantly less than commercial agencies. The cost-benefit analysis of employer-funded child care, commissioned by the Federal Government's Office of the Status of Women, argues that it is in a company's own commercial interest to provide work-place centres. Direct financial benefits are achieved through reduced labour turnover and absenteeism and substantial taxation concessions. There are also less quantifiable benefits in the form of improved worker morale, a better corporate image and industrial relations environment, and an improved ability to attract potential employees.

As more employers undertake to provide child care facilities, child care will be seen on a par with other general employee benefits, such as holiday pay, sick pay, and workers compensation. Once incorporated into the system, employment based child care will become increasingly difficult to disband. Employment based child care encourages workers. It not only validates women as mothers it also provides positive role modelling for children.

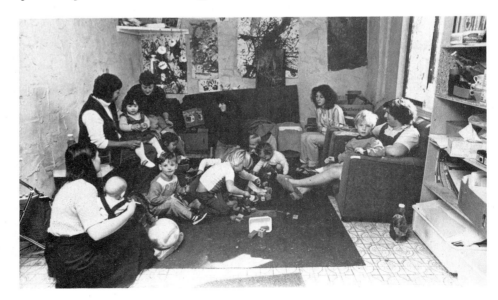

Child care is regarded by women as having as equal importance as wages

However, the fact that the mother is still tied to the children by physical proximity can have a negative effect on some mothers and children. This type of child care will always be controlled by employers and not by employees.

Locally based child care

Neighbourhood based child care is another option. This is often run by local women working together to provide child care services. This offers the power of networking and gives women power to determine the type of facilities they want. Children are with children from the same area and not dislocated out of their neighbourhood. However, it does include the negative aspects of two stop shopping and can be limited by the fact that the hours of many locally run child care centres often don't cater to the needs of mothers who do shift work.

Even when mothers attempt to provide adequate child care for their communities, they can be hampered by bureaucratic red tape. The Department of Family and Community Services is responsible for approving child care locations and places much emphasis on physical standards (see box p. 177).

WOMEN AND RETIREMENT

More and more, women are engaging in work outside the home, whether through financial necessity or personal choice. Yet alarmingly, very few women are making provision for their retirement. Under pressure from the superannuation industry, the Federal Government recently approved a major overhaul to superannuation legislation. One issue yet to be resolved concerns whether the retirement needs of women are addressed.

Cass, in her 1987 report to the federal government on retirement income policy, concluded that private superannuation should be available to those out of the workforce for long periods — such as women — and that contributions should be tax-deductible. Part-time workers, the majority of whom are women (80 per cent), are particularly disadvantaged. However, the superannuation case for all women is bleak. Of three million full-time female workers, only 46 per cent are covered by superannuation.

The economic security of women in their later years has a significant bearing on their health and independence (see chapter 14) This is an issue which needs to be addressed by women and employers alike and which has important ramifications for the future.

CASE STUDY

Cheryl was eighteen when her daughter, Belinda, was born. She had been so happy because she wanted her very badly. She had left school at sixteen — it had seemed pretty irrelevant then anyway — and she hadn't thought much about working. A baby of her own would give her security and a purpose in life.

Since Belinda turned three Cheryl has been a single parent.

Her daughter is now ten, and for the past two years they have been living in a small country town. After five years of battling in the inner city suburb in which she grew up, Cheryl

Super: women left out

Women are still not planning to be financially independent for their later years.

Even if they work part-time, as many do, women are unlikely to be covered by current super legislation.

At present, personal superannuation schemes which do not include employer contributions, do not allow contributions from temporarily unemployed workers.

Under pressure from the superannuation industry, the Federal Government recently approved a major overhaul to super legislation. There is concern that our increasingly aged population can no longer be supported by the Government pension system.

The focus of the review includes cover for public servants who have been previously excluded from any entitlement if they ceased working in their government job before the age of 55. As a result of the overhaul, it is likely that public servants will be able to retain the contributions made by the government if they move to other jobs.

But one issue yet to be resolved concerns the nature of women's work, and whether their retirement needs are being catered for.

Dr Bettina Cass, who was commissioned in 1987 by the Federal Government to review retirement income policy, has recently concluded that private superannuation should be available to those out of the workforce for long periods — such as women — and that contributions should be tax deductible.

The AMP Society has also recently commissioned a major study which found that part-time workers were suffering from the lack of access to superannuation.

Part-time workers in the main consist of women — of 1.5 million part-time workers in Australia, 80 per cent are women. Of three million full-time female workers, only 46 per cent are covered by superannuation.

According to the AMP Society study: 'Women are not planning actively for their own retirement despite the fact that there is every indication they should be.'

The superannuation industry itself is frustrated by the current legislation. Bain and Co's Ellie Fitz-Gerald says: 'The Government's clear aim must be to make us all self-sufficient in retirement. Surely as many obstacles as possible should be removed and encouragement given to those prepared to sacrifice their current cash flow for their own and the country's long term security.'

Particularly in the event of divorce, part of the husband's entitlements could be allocated to the wife to compensate for her contributions to the marital home.

According to Gina Baddely of Women's Investment Network (WIN), women who began a superannuation plan in the early years of their career now had the advantage of time on their side.

'One of our clients, a 27-year-old-nurse, began a financial plan two years ago. We decided that it would make more sense for her to concentrate on building a superannuation fund in the early years of her career because the money she accumulated would compound.

'If she paid $40 a week into superannuation for 10 years and made no further contributions, she could expect to retire at 55 with a payout of $800 000 compared with only $41 000 if she had begun contributing between the ages of 45 and 55.'

The calculation hinged on an annual return of 15.5pc, which WIN thinks is the overall average return of super funds.

Only 3 per cent of all Australian women depend on superannuation for their main source of retirement income.

Sally Fitzgerald, *Sun-Herald*, 23 July 1989.

decided to take control of her life by moving to a small town. She wanted to live without the constant stress of too little money, and too little time to meet the demands of working, mothering, and homemaking.

She purposely chose this town, because the food processing factory would provide work for her, and the environment would be healthier for Belinda. The weather was warm amd the distances were small enough that she could get by without a car. Cheryl found a job in the factory, and Belinda settled into school and made friends with whom she played after school. She shared after school care with other mothers, and certainly the financial pressures were less.

In spite of that, she soon came to hate the monotonous boredom of working as an impersonal part of a conveyor belt chain. Most afternoons she left the factory with a headache: the compounds used in the processing aggravating her hayfever, so that she was much more susceptible to sinus infections. Her wrists often ached as a result of the continuous repetitive movements on some parts of the chain, selecting and checking fruit. The managers tried to add variety to the work by changing the departments in which the women worked, but it did not help much.

On top of that, nearly all the other women had grown up in the region, they had husbands, children, parents, cousins and old friends in the area, and they didn't badly need to make new friends like Cheryl did. Many of them only worked in the factory part-time to supplement their incomes, they weren't absolutely dependent on it. Cheryl was angry that she had not been given better educational opportunities at school — the teachers always implied that the girls didn't really need to learn mathematics or science or read books. When she was fourteen she had known no better, but now she realised her double disadvantage. She was a woman without vocational skills, unable to increase her income, because she could not afford to retrain and support her daughter at the same time.

At the end of the first year she realised she was going to have to leave the factory because she now also suffered from dermatitis, and almost every afternoon she left the factory with a headache from the constant noise as well as her frequent episodes of hay fever and sinusitis.

She borrowed an old typewriter from Sophia who worked in the office, and had a daughter Belinda's age. For the next six months during evenings and weekends she taught herself to type. She was always so tired, she began to get impatient with Belinda, and sometimes felt she just could not take any more. If it hadn't been for the support and encouragement of Sophia she knew she could not have kept going. But she did, and she moved to an office job when one became available. That was six months ago.

Because of her experiences Cheryl has become more aware of the problems women encounter in their workplaces, and she has become angry that the factory management takes them for granted. She had never really thought about questions of rights and benefits before. Now she wants to know why the women process workers get no superannuation benefits and why there are no occupational health and safety services (the management even denies that the women may suffer from repetition strain injuries when working for hours using the same actions). Why are there no child care support services, which would help the women so much, when the factory is clearly dependent on them to keep production schedules up?

Since she and Sophia organised the visit of an equal opportunity officer recently, the women have discussed these matters a lot.

They now want Cheryl to lead a formal delegation to management to request better conditions for the women workers. Cheryl is undecided. At last she has a reasonably satisfying job, with enough money to keep herself and Belinda, and even has some time for recreation. What might be the risks, and what might be the benefits of leading the delegation? She will think about it and decide tonight...

References

Cass, B. (1988). *Review of retirement policy*, Department of Social Security, Canberra.

Herzog, M. (1972). *From hand to mouth: women and piecework*, Penguin, London.

Mathews, J. (1985). *Health and safety at work: a trade union's safety representatives handbook*, Pluto Press, Sydney.

National Women's Advisory Council (1983). *So much left undone, National Women's Advisory Council on disabled women and girls*, AGPS, Canberra.

National Women's Health Policy (1989). *National women's health policy: advancing women's health in Australia*, AGPS, Canberra.

NSW Anti-discrimination Board (1984). *Protective legislation at work — a case study of the 'weight limit' on manual handling*, A report of the President of the Anti-discrimination Board, NSW Anti-discrimination Board, Sydney.

Queensland Nurses Union of Employees (1986). *The incidence of back injuries within the Queensland nursing workforce 1981–1982 and 1984–1985*, Queensland Nurses Union, Brisbane.

Refshauge, C. (1986). *Interim report on protective provisions for manual handling: health and safety with equal employment opportunity*, Women's Bureau, Department of Employment and Industrial Relations.

Sivard, R.L. (1984). *Women ... a world survey*, World Priorities, Washington, D.C.

Women's Bureau, Department of Employment, Education and Training (1988). *Women at work — facts and figures*, Department of Employment, Education and Training, Canberra.

13 Women With Special Needs

This chapter explores the health of women with special needs. Four groups of women will be examined in detail: non English speaking background women, Aboriginal women, disabled women and rural women. For each group social disadvantage is acknowledged to have a significant effect on health outcomes. The inequities in access, control and appropriate service provision are exponentially compounded.

WOMEN FROM NON ENGLISH SPEAKING BACKGROUNDS

The Australian Bureau of Statistics (1982) reveals the following data on non English speaking background women:

- over two-thirds have no qualifications;
- 86.3 per cent have an annual income of less than $26,000; and
- they are more likely to be working as process workers (25 per cent) than in administration (1.6 per cent).

The social mores of non English speaking background women effect their ability to optimise health outcomes. Women from non English speaking backgrounds suffer from what Rohrbaugh (1979) termed 'triple exploitation'. They are female, a racial minority and more often poor. Rohrbaugh notes that in western countries more than two thirds of non English speaking background families are headed by women, and half of these families are below poverty level.

The National Migrant and Refugee Women Speak-Out on employment and health problems held in Sydney in 1982 identified three particular areas of concern in the health of non English speaking background women in Australia:

- the nature of migration;
- specific cultural health issues; and
- access to services.

Davis and George (1988) suggest that for non English speaking background women of many different cultural, linguistic and economic backgrounds, the relevant aspect of health status is their ability to gain access to the Australian health system. The development of an interpreter service, introduced in 1977, has improved communication and therefore access in hospitals. However 90 per cent of health care takes place in the community where only a limited telephone interpreting service is available.

The reasons for migration have an effect on health status and access of non English speaking background women to health services. Voluntary migration, i.e. where the decision to migrate is a woman's individual choice or a joint one between husband and wife, ensures that discordance over migration is not a contributor to poor health.

Immigration may be involuntary from the woman's point of view. For example, there are cases where migration is solely the husband's decision or where single women migrate to escape dowry payments or other family pressures. In such contexts, the translocation of these women from familiar contexts, combined with their isolation in inappropriate locations in a new country, may diminish their prospects of healthy lives.

The Better Health Commission (vol. 3) (1986) cited inequities in access to information, decision-making and the consultation process as barriers to the better health of non English speaking background women. The proposals suggested at the 1982 conference were echoed: more non English speaking background workers, health centres with bilingual health care workers, improved education of health providers, more interpreters, recognition of non English speaking background women's qualifications and national free medical scheme. In its 1987 Policy Statement, the NSW Department of Health's Migrant Health Division section lists 20 achievements in the area of migrant health. Only one relates directly to women:

> Bilingual Women's Community Educators Programme has been established in the Western and Southern Metropolitan Health Regions and Illawarra. This programme aims to provide health education and information programmes to non English speaking background women. (Ethnic Affairs Commission of NSW 1987).

The recommendations of the *National women's health policy* to improve access to health services for non English speaking background women were:

- additional health care interpreter services;
- special translator support services in homes for the aged; and
- extensive and regular use of ethnic media to inform these women about hospital and community services.

There are several specific health issues surrounding the health of non English speaking background women. These include reproductive issues such as contraception and family planning, mental and occupational health, and ageing.

The total aged ethnic population of Australia increased by 79 per cent during the 1970s, as opposed to a 25 per cent increase in the Australian born aged. As they age, non English speaking background women, as the *National women's health policy* states, are in 'triple jeopardy': women, older, and ethnic. Second language regression, i.e. the loss of English over time for those women who learnt English after arrival in Australia, is common. They are also in jeopardy because age and cultural differences prevent their full integration into Australian society. Their children, who often provide them with their only English lessons, have moved out and away. Hearst (1981) and Newman (1981) identify a demand for 'ethnic' nursing homes.

ABORIGINAL WOMEN

Sykes says of white doctors and black women

> many of the problems confronting Black women in the area of health could be considered problems not superficially related to their being women. However, the situation is that the responsibility for the health of the community generally lies in the hands of the women. Other, and equally important problems, such as unemployment, police/Black relations, and the heavy brunt of racist confrontation, tend to deploy the menfolk — leaving the everyday running of the house, family and community to the women. If there is to be any breakthrough by the medical profession in assisting the Black community to deal with its health problems on a day to day basis, this will mainly be actuated — if indeed it is actuated — through the women.

There are huge discrepancies in health status between the Aboriginal population and the rest of the Australian population. Even the available data is substandard. For example, maternal and infant mortality data for 1984 was available for only 35 per cent of the population. Health status indicators of the Aboriginal population in Australia resemble those of developing countries. For example, in New South Wales, the Aboriginal mortality rate is over four times higher than the state average. This inequity in health care is even more marked for Aboriginal women. The report of the Aboriginal Women's Task Force (1986) states that Aboriginal women 'not only are two to three times as likely to experience the trauma of an infant death, they can also expect to have a lifespan which is some twenty years shorter than that for non-Aboriginal women'.

The health of Aboriginal women is integral to the total well-being of Aboriginal communities. Flower (1987) believes that by 'lifting the standards of Aboriginal health in general, Aboriginal women's health will benefit immensely'.

Uwankara palyankyu kanyintjaku

The Anangu Pitjantjatjara (pronounced Pit'n-jara) live in the remote area that crosses the state borders of South Australia, Western Australia and the Northern Territory, and their lands cover about one-tenth of South Australia. Since gaining land rights in 1981, increasing numbers of anangu (the Pitjantjatjara word for people) are returning to their original land, only travelling to the more established communities to visit relatives, to shop, to attend the health clinic or to have their say in community management meetings.

By the mid-1980s, the anangu knew they had a very great health care problem. The children in these communities were eighty times more likely than their white counterparts to suffer from pneumonia; in 1985 each person visited the clinic or hospital over 18 times per year, on average.

The anangu realised that they needed more than band-aid therapeutics, that their poor diets and poor housing contributed significantly to their health problems. In 1983, after years of negotiations with authorities, Anangu Pitjantjatjara (AP) started its own community-controlled health service, the Nganampa Health Council. In a statement about the aims of the council, its chair, Yami Lester, said: 'The health service will be looking after the health of all the people, not just sickness, but how to keep well and strong.'

In early 1986, the council decided to undertake a detailed survey of the entire AP lands as part of a major review of the public and environmental health situation. The review would try to avoid some of the problems of earlier assessments by involving local communities and emphasising the role of local people and communities in managing their own affairs.

The review, which was called *Uwankara Palyankyu Kanyintjaku* (or *A Strategy for Well Being*) discovered that only about half of the population actually lived in houses. Over half the houses had major malfunctions such as raw sewage floating in the living areas or exposed electrical wiring which actually turned the houses into health hazards. It was clear that housing needed to be used as a way of addressing the complex inter-relationships of health and living conditions. For example, food storage and preparation should be a health-promoting activity which takes place in a house, yet for anangu food storage is such a problem that most families buy their food daily, or even twice daily, if they can afford to do so, and food preparation mostly means cooking over the outside fire in a single pot or frying pan.

During the review, it was agreed that local responsibility for repairs and maintenance could work only if there was a sufficient standard applied for building houses, for supervising work and, possibly most importantly, for coordinating the activities of the enormous range of funding and implementing agencies which were used to dealing with individuals and small communities on an ad hoc basis. One community reported that it had been called to 142 community meetings over a three-month period by a plethora of outside agencies.

Something as simple as washing children shows the problems that existed in the communities. Parents are understandably unwilling to wash their children in winter without hot water, and in many houses there is no water at all. Even though anangu may have been 'given' health education about good hygiene, the knowledge could not be used.

'Essential health hardware' also includes sewage and drainage, taps that work, and rubbish disposal. While these are all basic things which most of us take for granted and have immediately repaired if they break, this has not been the case in the majority of Aboriginal communities. Camp dogs also contribute to disease among children by spreading hepatitis B, scabies, fleas and other infections.

Until now, there has not been a well-developed structure of local and regional management to deal with the maintenance of houses. This problem has been exacerbated by the poor coordination of housing projects, with a number of different departments and agencies contributing to different stages. Supervision of contractors has been poor, allowing some to perform sub-standard work. The review recommended that the AP council and the Nganampa Health Council take over major responsibility for coordinating inputs.

One of the most significant outcomes of the review was an agreement by a major funding body, the Aboriginal Development Corporation, to fund maintenance which involved either safety or critical health hardware problems, while leaving the local communities to look after the less urgent issues. This involves a major improvement in community and regional management, with an easily implemented system for notification of problems.

A number of community councils have shifted their management focus to improving the living conditions of their community members. This entails the monitoring and prompt repair — resources permitting — of housing problems, more systematic rubbish collection, a tree planting program, and firewood collection. Desperately needed are two plumbers and two electricians to work across the land; unfortunately, funding for these falls into a bureaucratic no man's land.

Another significant outcome of the report was the opening of a public health office at the Nganampa Health Council, with responsibility for supervising the public and environmental health of the people in the lands. This fits in well with the general community feeling that it was time to do something more to improve health status.

According to Yami Lester the implementation of the report is progressing very well. A significant component of the implementation rests on reporting back to the community the findings of the survey, together with suggestions of how the community can bring about change using its own resources. For the first time, local stores have started to talk to the health clinics, schools and to the community managers about improving the quality of food available to the community — particularly important in view of the rising prevalence of diabetes and the discovery that average daily consumption of sugar was equivalent to 66 teaspoons — excluding soft drinks.

The report and the model it espouses have been recommended for an award from the World Health Organisation, and other Aboriginal communities are starting to pick up some the ideas.

Lewis Kaplan, *Australian Society*, February 1990.

The report of the Aboriginal Women's Task Force identified three areas of concern for the health of Aboriginal women:

- the paucity of Aboriginal health care workers;
- reproductive issues, particularly maternal and infant mortality; and
- violence.

In the 1980s Aboriginal women have taken a leading role in helping to shape change in the area of Aboriginal health. For example, in the Northern Territory they far outnumber men as health care providers. In the same state, as health care consumers, Aboriginal women act as community advocates, e.g. The Alice Springs Birth Rights Project (the Congress Alukura). The role of these women Aboriginal health workers is often one of mediating between traditional and western medicine.

Particularly where reproductive issues are concerned, the health of Aboriginal women has deteriorated through the forced breakdown of the Aboriginal culture. The dispersal of Aborigines into settlements and the separation from their children has resulted in a loss of the traditional means of disseminating information about sex to younger generations. The Aboriginal Task Force concluded that many Aboriginal women remained 'ignorant of the basic facts about sex matters and without control over this aspect of their lives which leaves them particularly vulnerable to sexual exploitation and victimisation.'

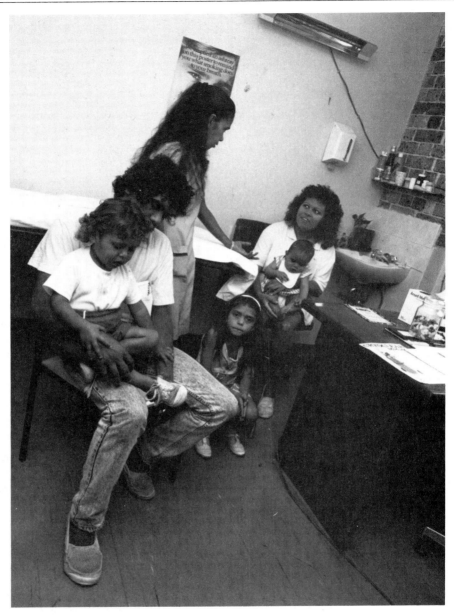

The Aboriginal Medical Service in Redfern, Sydney

In the area of contraception, debate has raged over the use of long acting injectable contraceptives, e.g. Depo Provera, for Aboriginal women. The NSW Aboriginal Medical Service has called for an active campaign to stop its use, while state Family Planning Associations are permitted limited prescribing rights.

For many Aboriginal women, going to the doctor is a stressful experience. The Task Force reported that many Aboriginal women avoid consulting a doctor on their own behalf, particularly concerning abdominal or sexual complaints, as Sykes illustrates:

> A difference of opinion also exists in regard to intimate personal examination by a young male doctor of a Black woman. While it is fairly acceptable practice in the white community for a white male doctor to carry out intimate examinations of white females on a first visit, such practice is — to some sections of the Black community — totally unacceptable. Even to Black women who might otherwise be amenable to the idea in different circumstances, in what may be regarded by her as a hostile environment she is likely to view the experience — or even the notion — as traumatic. With very few exceptions, Black women avoid consulting a doctor on their own behalf especially in regard to abdominal or sexual complaints.

This may also be a contributing factor to high infant mortality rates, as Aboriginal women avoid antenatal visits. Transportation to medical services and accommodation at hospitals also provide problems.

Surgery, too, can be seen as cause for great anxiety. Reid (1978) found this in her study of an Aboriginal community in the Northern Territory.

> The attitudes of community members towards surgery, then, derive from the collective convictions that it is fraught with risk, that it is an unnatural assault on the integrity of the body, that it will weaken the patient through loss of blood and that it resembles the methods of the sorcerer. These attitudes are shared almost equally by young and old. They are but one enduring aspect of an indigenous system of beliefs about the body, social and political relations, and the nature of powers of the sacred world which are an integral part of the world view of the people of northeastern Arnhem Land.

Aboriginal women have suffered from both rape and domestic violence. Rape and physical abuse of Aboriginal women by white men characterised the early white colonisation of Australia. 'Gin sprees' where the object of the event was to rape, maim or kill as many black women as possible, were common. More recently, alcohol abuse has led to increased violence against Aboriginal women.

WOMEN IN RURAL AND REMOTE AREAS

The basis of rural women's health problems requires an understanding of the socio-demographic issues which affect the lives of these women, e.g. their lack of power and control over natural wealth and resources and their physical and emotional isolation. Major factors include:

- low incomes;
- hazardous occupations, e.g. rural textile workers, the majority of whom are women, are surrounded by cotton dust and asbestos;
- lower than average educational level, which traditionally has correlated with poor usage of health services; and
- a proportionally higher number of elderly women and young children in rural areas.

Environmental factors are also significant, e.g. many rural homes, especially within Aboriginal settlements, do not have clean water or adequate sewage. Public transportation systems are also limited, thereby restricting women's access to health care services.

Access is only one of many problems in health service provision to women in rural areas. A maldistribution of doctors and medical services exists between urban and rural communities. For example, the overall general practitioner/patient ratio in New South Wales is approximately 1:900. Some rural areas have a ratio of 1:3000. The *National women's health policy* cites the difficulties of low income women in small country towns:

- in some one-doctor towns fee for service at time of consultation can effectively deny access to medical treatment and where there is no Medicare office there is no ability to claim immediate reimbursement of the rebate;
- a lack of privacy in isolated areas, particularly in company towns;
- the lack of choice of doctor and sex of doctor.

The inequality in the number of doctors in rural areas obscures other problems, e.g. the needs of rural women in the areas of family planning and prevention of breast and cervical cancer are not addressed. Moreover, country women often must travel to the city if they are seeking a termination of their pregnancy. In response to the needs of rural and remote area women to appropriate gynaecological services, women's health nurses were trained to provide these services in particular rural areas.

The introduction of women's health nurses is an important step in addressing the unmet health needs of rural women. Unfortunately the introduction of these nurses has met with mixed response from both the general practitioners and the communities. The screening and preventive tasks of these nurses have not been linked to the conventional treatment and curative processes. Although the initiative is still relatively new, it seems that a fragmented service has replaced an inadequate one.

DISABLED WOMEN

Segan (1980) suggests that there are both negative and positive interactive effects unique to disabled women. The negative aspects include:

- the norm of passivity that is a feature of many special needs groups;
- the perception of physical imperfection; and
- the myth of asexuality.

The positive features include:

- the ability to regard able bodyism as restrictive and narrow, from which follows the ability to dress comfortably and be accepted as a friend; and
- the ability to develop and maintain strong family ties with parents and siblings.

The 'disabled' often now use the term 'differently abled' to reinforce the positive aspects. Becker (1978) summarises the struggle in the following way 'we are the first and foremost sensitive human beings with a terrific sense of accomplishment after all of the horrible but challenging experiences we have been through'.

Fine and Asch (1988) suggest that there is very little recent data available relating to the extent and experience of disability in the population at large, particularly amongst women. The 1981 Australian Bureau of Statistics survey of handicapped people in Australia found that:

- equal numbers of handicapped men and women live in the community;
- women made up two-thirds of the handicapped living in institutions; and
- women represent 58.5 per cent of the severely handicapped.

Educational and occupational disadvantage is a recurring theme for women. O'Toole and Weeks (1978) cite a United States Government Report published in 1976 which noted that:

- disabled men were more likely to receive vocational, school and on the job training;
- a higher percentage of disabled men, 93.1 per cent were rehabilitated into wage-earning occupations (compared with 68.5 per cent of disabled women);
- the average weekly earnings for disabled men after rehabilitation were significantly higher than for women;
- disabled men were located in a wider range of occupations whilst women were clustered in a few areas (services, clerical).

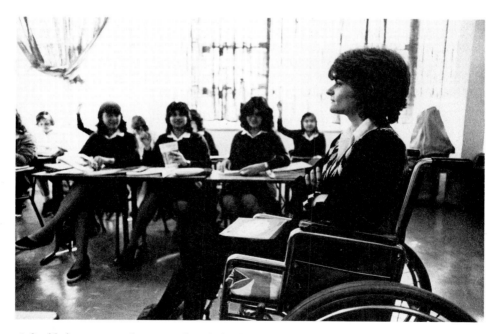

A disabled woman teacher at a Sydney high school

Steinberg (1983) in her special consultations with disabled women and girls in Australia found that they also had difficulties with employment. Steinberg's study cited employment status as a major problem for 30 per cent of the respondents. Access, accommodation and finances were other issues mentioned by Steinberg. She noted that the most effective long term support for these disabled women was provided by family and friends. The primary methodology of Steinberg's study involved a phone-in. Women with intellectual speech or hearing disabilities who were less likely to respond were encouraged to respond in writing.

Australian Bureau of Statistics (1988) data reveal that assistance with the tasks of daily living was also a substantial problem for women. Across all age groups a greater percentage of disabled women were found to need help compared to men. For example, in the age range five to 75 and over, 60 per cent of women need help compared to 40 per cent of men. The most frequently reported needs were for assistance with home maintenance, household domestic work and transport.

The need for rehabilitation of disabled women has not been widely explored. Ward (1989) suggests that the Commonwealth Rehabilitation Service, established in 1948 emphasised rehabilitation of the war wounded or work injured person — invariably a male. She found that rehabilitation services for disabled women were less than optimum. In studying the referral of women who sustained closed head injuries to a Commonwealth Rehabilitation Service, Ward found that the average length of time from injury until referral was 1.8 years. Only 12.5 per cent of all women who were referred to the service came directly from a State hospital program.

CASE STUDY

Liz felt as though she was a juggler in a circus act, trying to keep track of several things at once, and to keep them all in balance with one another.

The meeting had already been going on for nearly an hour, with different participants each wanting to make their points. It had been called to allow representatives of migrant women's groups to give feedback to the State Government about its new migrant health service guidelines for menopausal women.

Liz was a regional advisor for women's affairs, and although she had an educational background, women's health was one of her main areas of interest. Thus she had been asked to chair this meeting.

The problem was that the new guidelines, suggested that non English speaking background women required specially formulated programs for each group. While Liz didn't disagree with the guidelines, the interpretation of them by planners and health professionals, who were unfamiliar with educational and health promotion priniciples, led to confusion both amongst themselves, and in many consumer groups. Today's meeting was an example of this.

'Perhaps I can summarise the discussion of the last hour, before we move to other issues', she suggested.

'Representatives are here of the seven major ethnic groups in our region. While everybody agrees that accessibility to health services is a problem, we each see the problem from a different perspective. However, three aspects keep coming up — these are to do with barriers because of language difficulties, barriers due to cultural differences, and thirdly practical barriers of transport and language which discourage many women from using the available services'.

'Yet, when we explore the issue more, the balance and importance of these is different in each of the groups.

On the other hand the Area Health Services are trying to provide relevant services within the amount of money that is available. It seems that while physiological processes are the same, the cultural and symbolic connotations of menopause are different in different groups'.

'Thus our task as professional health planners is to provide a process of developing services; while the task of each ethnic group is to supply information, advice, and opinions so that a viable service can be placed within a given framework. If we look at it this way, we can see why some confusion has developed about whether the services will be similar or different. They'll be similar in some ways and different in others'.

'Can we carry on now and see whether there are any common priority areas which we could explore a little more to see if, in fact, you agree with my interpretation....'

REFERENCES

Australian Bureau of Statistics (1981). *Survey of handicapped persons, Australia*, ABS, Canberra, Cat. no. 4343.0.

Australian Bureau of Statistics (1982). *Family survey: Australian families*, ABS, Canberra, Cat. No. 4408.0.

Becker, E.F. (1978). *Female sexuality following spinal cord injury*, Chaever, Bloomington.

Better Health Commission (1986). *Looking forward to better health*, vol. 3, AGPS, Canberra.

Davis, A. & George, J. (1988). *States of health: health and illness in Australia*, Harper & Row, Sydney.

Ethnic Affairs Commission of NSW (1987). *Review of the ethnic affairs policy statements (EAPS) program in New South Wales*, Ethnic Affairs Commission of NSW, Sydney.

Fine, M. & Asch, A. (eds) (1988). *Women with disabilities — essays in psychology, culture and politics*, Temple University Press, Philadelphia.

Flower, D. (1987). *The Aboriginal health worker*, Vol ii, No 2.

Hearst, S. (1981). *Ethnic communities and their aged*, Clearing House on Migration Issues, Carlton.

National Women's Health Policy (1989). *National women's health policy: advancing women's health in Australia*, AGPS, Canberra.

Newman, R. (ed.) (1981). *Ageing migrants in Australia — planning towards 1985*, New South Wales Council on the Ageing, Sydney.

O'Toole, J.C. & Weeks, C. (1978). *What happened after school? A study of disabled women's education equity*, Communications Network Far West Laboratory for Educational Research and Development, San Francisco.

Reid, J. (1978). The dangers of surgery: an Aboriginal view, *The medical journal of Australia*, 1, 90–92.

Rohrbaugh, J.B. (1979). *Women: psychology's puzzle*, Basic Books, New York.

Segan, L. (1980). Sexuality and the mentally handicapped and sexuality and the physically handicapped, *New doctor*, 17, October.

Steinberg, M. (1983). *Special consultations with disabled women and girls*, National Women's Advisory Council Research Report.

Sykes, B. (1980). White doctors and black women, *New doctor*, 15, 33–35.

Ward, D. (1989). *Equity in access and provision of service for women with a disability*, Unpublished paper.

14 Women and Ageing

The health problems of women as they age are many. They relate to the decline in socio-economic status that women undergo, inhibiting their access to services. These services, when they are available, are often inappropriate. Current definitions of ageing have led to a medicalisation of the ageing process for women — decline in function is treated medically which leads to alienation and dependence. Strategies to reorientate the negative aspects of ageing for women include increasing their involvement in their own health care and redirecting the focus on ageing from the burden of illness to the development of health as an outcome.

DEFINITIONS OF OLD AGE

Throughout history, societies have struggled with the definition of old age. Hippocrates (460 – 377 BC) referred to old age as the 'age of winter'. In the latter half of the twentieth century the definitions are less romantic and more numeric. In 1981, Anderson was still using the World Health Organisation's numeric classification for older persons developed in 1963:

- middle aged 45–59;
- elderly 60–74;
- old 75–89; and
- very old from 90 years on.

In 1985, the United Nations sought to refine this definition in its *International glossary of social gerontology*. However, as populations age, particularly in the western world, any numeric definition of older persons is under potential review. Lesnoff-Caravaglia and Klys (1987) argue that a meaningful framework for the discussion of aged subgroups should commence at age 70 years.

The societal definition of older persons includes a component related to employment. Retirement age can define numeric old age. In Australia, retirement is synonymous with eligibility for the old age pension, i.e. 60 years of age for women and 65 years for men. This definition of retirement is dependent on two erroneous assumptions about women in the workforce. The first is that although women live on average for five years more than men, they cannot work for as many years as men, hence the retirement age five years younger than men. The second assumption is that women are sicker than men and therefore will be unable to work their full quota of years to 65. Retiring women earlier than men has profound implications for their health. The old age pension cannot match the income these women received whilst working. Often they have outlived their male partners. They are financially disadvantaged and their socio-economic status lowers. Not only is their access to health care services made more difficult but also poverty related health problems such as inadequate diet and dentition are accentuated.

Another financial benchmark for measuring age has been superannuation, which is currently available to some workers at 55 years of age. Thus, while the lifespan of women is increasing, their working life is decreasing. Even when employer initiated superannuation is mandatory, such as in the Public Service, it holds little promise of economic and therefore health security for working women. Reproductive commitments often mean that women are not in the workforce long enough to qualify for employer contributions to superannuation. Women relying on superannuation in their retirement can expect to live for at least 20 years on an income fixed early in their working lives (see chapter twelve).

A method of bypassing the conflicts of defining old age numerically or by work is to relate old age to disability. This process serves to free older people from the stereotypes that govern numeric age. Disability may be a marker of the older individual. A whole new range of definitions emerge, some with negative associations, e.g. Hicks (1986) terminology of the 'frail elderly' and the 'not so frail elderly' and Lesnoff-Caravaglia and Klys's (1987) comical definitions of the 'frisky' and the 'risky'. However, most of these definitions relate to the inability of men to perform their work tasks. As definitions of older age for women they may be inappropriate.

Biological definition

According to 1988 statistics from the Commonwealth Department of Community Services and Health, the ageing population is the major consumer of health care services and resources in Australia.

Unfortunately these data rely on a biological definition of what constitutes the ageing population which encompasses the ideas of loss of organ reserve and capacity e.g. organs, like ovaries cannot function properly. This type of definition of loss reinforces the notion that women are reproductive vessels and when this part of their life has ended so has their main function.

The implication is that once women lose their menses they have lost their function in society. It is also at this time that their families are separating and reproducing. So not only do menopausal women feel an acute sense of loss of their baby-bearing potential, they are also losing their mothering role.

Some women, however, don't see the absence of menses as a loss. Rather, they experience relief. They no longer need to focus on the monthly activities of their uterus, nor do they have to worry about becoming pregnant in middle age. In this way, menopause is seen as a transition for women into a new phase of their lives, freeing them from the burdens of reproduction and enabling them to explore their needs as a woman, not just as a mother (see chapters six and seven).

Other losses cannot so easily become positive experiences. The senses decline with age. Vision can be affected in many ways. As the bones of the body grow old and brittle, the bones of the ear degenerate and hearing becomes impaired. The Australian government subsidises hearing aids in the older community, but once again, priorities are directed towards the younger population and workers and there are long waiting lists.

Diminished sense of the position of the joints, which occurs with ageing, often results in a loss of stability, so falls are common. Mineral depleted long bones of older women are more often broken, particularly the hip and the forearm, usually caused by stretching out the arm to prevent an impending fall. Recovery is slowed with old age and often it is incomplete, with some residual loss of function, particularly at hinge joints such as the elbow and knee. The aim of rehabilitation of older women is usually to return them to the lifestyle from which they came. Hence their need for optimal function is not as great as would be needed by a worker. The accepted level of residual disability is far greater for women.

SOCIAL ASPECTS OF AGEING

In western cultures, older women, particularly those in retirement, become separated from the routines of social exchange. Both Johnson (1975) and Mauss (1954) maintain that older women, after their reproductive duties are completed, are shifted from the centre of social life in middle age to the periphery in old age. As Mauss (1954) identified in his concept of the gift relationship, older persons no longer participate in the giving of products, only in the receiving:

- the pension;
- superannuation; and
- health care.

The gift relationship is unbalanced. In traditional cultures, the balance of the gift relationship is maintained, with older women playing an important role. Often, they are responsible for supporting and maintaining family systems, e.g. through child care, education and rites of passage.

There are other ways of looking at ageing which are more conducive to women. As both McPherson-Turner (1980) and Webster (1980) point out, ageing can be seen as a natural progression of continuous growth and adaptation, rather than as a expression of continuous decline. Maggie Kuhn (1977), one of the founders of

The mid-life transition for the home-maker

Only two generations ago the average woman was in her fifties when her last child left home; she had little experience outside of her homemaking activities, her life was defined by the needs of her family. She was fast approaching old age and the prospects of widowhood, possible poverty and death.

Today she is in her forties, she is fit and healthy, she is economically stable and has a reasonable level of education, or even an established career. She has thirty or forty good years ahead. She is ready for a new lease of life.

Many of these women embrace middle age with excitement. They have raised their children, they have worked part-time to help clear the mortgage, they have supported the careers or business pursuits of their husbands.

'Now it's my turn!'

Having invested much of their lives in the development of loved ones, they are excited by the prospect of self-development. Perhaps for the first time they may feel free to pursue a self-directed path in life, something that men often take for granted but which most married women with children find impossible to achieve, or if they do, it is often with a sense of guilt.

This is the happiest scenario for the married woman whose children have grown up. Yet even so she is likely to find opposition — her husband and children may be reluctant to surrender their hold on her, she has always been there for them and they may baulk at fending for themselves.

Some middle-aged husbands may be willing to start sharing the cooking and the laundry and the shopping, others will be dismayed at the prospect.

When husbands are more dismayed and threatened than excited by the new development of their wives, then trouble can occur.

There is a peak in the divorce rate at around 25 years of marriage and much of this reflects the struggle for a wife to liberate herself from the constraints of family life against the steady opposition of a husband who may not see the potential for a new and better life.

Many husbands are puzzled by this period of adjustment, and wonder whether it is indeed some form of menopausal madness.

They may be bewildered by protests such as:

I want to be a real person
I want some freedom
I want some space
I want to find out who I am

The bemused husband asks:

Hasn't she always been free to do what she wants?
Hasn't she had time and money available to do this?
Hasn't she had freedom?

If he has felt forced to struggle in the rat race day after day, locked into mortgage repayments and family and job obligations, experiencing precious little sense of personal freedom, he may have looked at her life as being relatively free and his own as being more of a prison or a trap.

What husbands and wives seldom understand is that each of us may be living in a prison of sorts and that these prisons often exist within ourselves. Sex roles and life scripts are two sorts of prisons.

It may be a woman's own definition of womanhood, her own view of what a good wife and mother should be that is most imprisoning for her. These internal expectations are known as sex role stereotypes, they are like internalised blueprints or computer programs with instructions or printouts on:

How to be a woman
How to be a man

We develop these blueprints from birth onwards and they are determined not only by what our parents teach us but by what we see and hear around us in our particular cultures, and what we read and observe via the mass media.

For example a woman's stereotypes may include:

People will think I'm a bad wife if I don't cook a nice meal every evening.
My husband will think I'm a bad wife if I don't cook a nice meal every evening.

This may be an implicit and firm belief within her and she may comply faithfully with this belief, never so much as questioning it in her own mind, let alone challenging the assumption in her family. Then after 20 or 30 years of this sort of dedicated behaviour, she may start to question and perhaps to resent some of her duties to others. She may come to ask herself why she should spend hours each day preparing meals and why she shouldn't sometimes decide on different priorities. If she believes that these are her obligations to her family and that these obligations are cast in stone and can never be renegotiated, then she is likely to feel resentful and trapped. Perhaps she comes to feel tyrannised by family obligations and then she begins to feel that the tyranny is being imposed upon her by her husband and family. Her husband and family may well expect these things — it has always been this way, why should it be any different?

In many cases these expectations have never been questioned, and often no thought has been given to the possibility of renegotiation. Frequently there is some expectation that the outcome will be disastrous if we do not stick to our blueprints.

But how catastrophic will the consequences be if we fail to meet these implicit expectations?

More often it is the assumption that the consequences will be hideous that stops us from challenging expectations. What if you don't cook every evening? He'll be surprised and disappointed, certainly. He may even be angry and disapproving. Don't expect him to congratulate you. But will he stop loving you? Will he abandon you? Will he attack you?

It is just possible, of course, that he might do any of these things, but it is even more likely that he will recover from the shock of domestic revolution and that he will adjust. After all he has had to adjust to many other dramatic changes and disappointments in his life, as all mature adults do.

Many women who experience a great resistance in the family to any change in their behaviour complain that their husbands are like children and expect to be cared for like children, and these women often become very bitter and resentful. Yet it is important to realise that if you insist upon catering to his every need, then you are encouraging him to behave like a child.

One of the most common husband-wife conflicts that is likely to erupt at this time is a result of each spouse taking up an accusatory position with the other. A wife may feel that her husband is responsible for her unhappiness:

he has oppressed her;
he has taken her for granted;
he has made her a slave to him and the children;
he has insisted that she follow him and his work opportunities wherever they have taken him.

In response to these accusations a husband will feel bewildered and angry. Often he has been faithfully obeying the stereotype or blueprint for what constitutes a good husband and provider and he does not see himself as a tyrant or bully. He will respond with a counter attack:

she is hysterical and demanding and unreasonable;
she is vacillating and never able to decide what she wants;
she is more interested in the opinions of her mother, friends, therapist, than in his.

This sort of interchange rapidly escalates to the point of marital schism.

The lines are drawn, now they are enemies. In her eyes he has proven himself to be uncaring, unfeeling, selfish and undermining of her. He sees her becoming distraught and regards her response as irrational and hysterical.

All of this might be avoided if the two can consider that whatever harm they may have caused each other may have been done in ignorance rather than in malice, that the sense of imprisonment is often mutual, and that both of them may profit from escape. He may have taken her for granted, but she might have made herself endlessly available to him.

She might have seemed too involved with her mother, sister, friends, but perhaps it has been easier for him to accept this rather than to struggle to understand her and to communicate with her.

If this wife can explain to her husband how she has allowed the expectations of others to dominate her life, he may listen and he may understand. He is less likely to listen if she accuses him of imprisoning her with his demands and expectations.

Our expectations of ourselves are constructed in very complicated ways, and they include:

what I expect me to be

what he expects me to be (or, rather, what I believe he expects of me, which may not be the same thing, and which I may never discover if we have never communicated clearly with each other).

Then there are the expectations I have grown up with — what my mother and father expect of me, what they have demonstrated to me as role models, the sort of life they have encouraged me to develop, the values they have passed on.

If our mothers have taught us to have little separate identity and to subsume ourselves to the service of others, then it may be that they have only repeated to us the message that was passed on to them.

If they have taught us only how to achieve our ends by manipulations rather than by direct assertion, then we must understand that our mothers, like ourselves, had few alternative role models.

If a wife can explain to her husband how she has come to challenge some of the stereotypes and how she has come to feel tyrannised by them, then perhaps she can encourage him to look at his own imprisonment. Without the focus of accusation and blame, men and women can help each other because they have different abilities and strengths.

Some men will feel just as imprisoned by the cultural expectations of machoism and may welcome the opportunity to break out. Those who will not break out may be acting out of fear rather than spitefulness. Prisoners who are liberated after many years of imprisonment often want to return to prison. The freedom is too terrifying.

For the wife who believes that her husband is resisting her liberation just because he does not want to compromise his own life style, there may be a need for complex negotiation and, ultimately, confrontation.

As well, we must confront our own behaviours.

If you have been a willing servant to your family, then you cannot entirely blame your husband or your children or your mother (who probably taught you how to be a domestic slave). But neither should you blame yourself. The emancipation of women has been one of the greatest revolutions of our time, bringing with it upheaval and confusion and new problems, but also new opportunities.

This revolution in the role of women and in the relationships between men and women poses enormous difficulties for us all, but women are renowned for their endurance, for their skillful communication and for their sensitivity to the feelings and needs of others. These feminine characteristics will stand them in good stead. They will gain the understandings of others by patient, skillful, sensitive negotiation — this is the feminine way.

Carolyn Quadrio

Greypower, has tried to address this by making her definitions powerful and non-sexist. She identifies three ways for older women to become empowered by ageing:

- speaking your own mind;
- outliving your opposition; and
- integrating your knowledge and experience with the energy of the young.

She goes on to discuss other concepts/values which recognise the positive experiences of ageing:

- survival and capacity to cope with change;
- the ability to test new lifestyles without the need to compete with existing structures; and,
- the coalition of groups joined by the universalising factor of ageing.

She describes the aged as the enablers, energisers and liberators in society.

Women friends and relatives are expected to care for each other and wait on their partners. Studies of carers of older persons in Australia, 90 per cent of whom are women, show that these women see themselves as workers, providing unpaid services to their aged relatives. This overwhelming attention to physical decline of others imprisons the carers. Kinnear and Graycar (1982) concluded in their study of carers that a marked deterioration had occurred in many important areas of the carers lifestyle. Problems encountered included a deterioration in their relationships with their husbands, an inability to sleep and a fear about growing older.

In Braithwaite's (1986) study, 73 per cent of carers were not prepared to leave the person they were caring for alone. The carers would only allow themselves to be temporarily relieved by assistance from alternate carers, usually friends, relatives or health care providers. Philips (1984) argues that perpetuating the unpaid work of women into older age is tacitly supported by governments who see this care as a way of saving money.

Twenty years of preparing for widowhood

My father spent more than 20 years preparing my mother for widowhood. In fact, from the time of his first massive heart attack he felt a responsibility to prepare mum for his death. He was a doctor (so was she) and I suppose he encountered many widows and few widowers in his practice. His heart must have gone out to all those widows he saw failing to cope.

Certainly, when I chose as a life partner a man seven years my junior, I had the feeling dad was happy with the age gap — so we would 'go together' or relatively closely together and I wouldn't be left to cope on my own.

How did dad prepare mum for widowhood? In three main ways, that I recall. Firstly, he kept his own affairs in scrupulous order. He had a filing cabinet and a filing system that were impressive for their clarity and accessibility. Great big labels written in black block letters — 'CAR INSURANCE', 'BANK SAFETY DEPOSIT BOX', 'WILL' — graced each suspension file.

He even had a small notebook with an alphabetical index which explained and clarified the filing system, indeed duplicated it in microcosm so that target files could be hunted down first in the notebook and then tracked to the filing cabinet. Rather like a library — easy, clear, effortless, foolproof, mumproof.

Once, when they were overseas and had left all their affairs in my hands, I actually had to use the little notebook to find an important document. So clear and easy were the instructions that I found what I was looking for in a flash. He prepared all this for mum so that she could cope without him.

Secondly, there were the 'banking sessions' on winter evenings. I remember mum, in her yellow woolly jumper with the brass buttons, sitting in the kitchen, listening patiently to dad while he explained terms such as 'withdrawal', 'deposit' and which accounts were which and which forms went with which accounts.

Mum looked like she was trying to seem interested and show respect for the individualised training she was being given, but there was a faint larrikin glint in her eye, something that suggested that she was attending but not storing. The fact that these sessions were repeated, identically, at various intervals through the year and over the years, testifies to the fact that little indeed was stored.

Thirdly, as a fall-back, fail-safe device, dad kept us children — mainly me — aware of all his affairs so that we would be totally dependable in a crisis, that is, in the event of his death.

Her welfare, her ability to cope without him, was his abiding concern through those 20-odd years and as I recall his devotion, it endears him to me even more. Once, I forget which heart attack it was, when he had good reason to believe that the next 12 hours would be his last, he called me to his bedside and extracted from me the vow that 'no matter what, I would look after mum'.

His health, I suppose, was broken first by the war in Eastern Europe, then by post-war refugee stress as he and mum struggled to pick up the threads of their lives and start over — new land, new freedom, new life.

He had his first attack in his 50s. I've lost track of how many followed. The call in the night, the ambulance, the flashing light in the dark street, the stretcher, the oxygen tanks and morphine injections, all blend into one. I've lost count, too, of the number of times I have said goodbye to him in my head.

Each time, each crisis, mum took over. Like a military reserve unit. She came out of herself. His time of weakness became her time of strength.

Suddenly she had energy, strength, commitment, direction, confidence and even a sense of humour — all the things she lacked when things were going well in our family. Sometimes dad would joke that his death would be her blossoming.

But it was never more than a joke. He continued to worry about how she would cope. Every widow whose loneliness or ineptitude he witnessed seemed to strengthen his own resolve.

Then in his late 60s, he had a heart bypass operation that turned his life inside out. Angina, that constant companion, disappeared. He was a model patient, keeping to a diet and an exercise routine and he fared well. Despite the odd hiccup, which he accepted as part of the package, today he is a walking testimony to the wonders of medical technology and his own indomitable will to live.

As for mum, it didn't come quickly. We saw it approach from afar. At first, like a storm in the distance, then the clouds came closer and we saw her gradual deterioration.

Suddenly, the storm was upon us and we lived through the relentless phases of her demise until one day, nearly three years ago, with dad by her side and her children in the wings, slowly and almost with dignity, she died.

Ruth Wajnryb, *Sydney Morning Herald*, May 7 1990.

As women grow older and outlive their partners and social supports, their isolation from the community increases. They are often alienated from making important decisions about their lives, e.g. choices regarding social interactions. They often end up in publicly funded institutional care, retirement villages, nursing homes, boarding houses and hostels.

OLDER WOMEN AND THE HEALTH CARE SYSTEM

Forecasts for the 21st century indicate that the proportion of women over 65 in the population will continue to increase. Women currently comprise 58 per cent of the over 65 years age group and 63 per cent of the over 75 years age group (ABS 1982).

The combination of old age and sickness will increasingly apply to women. The Australian Institute of Health (1988) in its report found that reporting of acute and chronic symptoms increased with age. Approximately 80 per cent of women aged 60 years or more said that they had at least one chronic illness.

Access to health care becomes a problem. Australia has a national health insurance scheme which covers all Australians through a taxation levy (Medicare). However, the services provided in certain key areas of decline for older women e.g. dentistry, orthopaedics, ophthalmology and otolaryngology are essentially private and expensive. Thus women's access to these services is hampered. As a result, older women are disadvantaged financially in their ability to avail themselves of health care services.

The majority of older women do not work long enough to qualify for any benefits such as superannuation. Most are financially dependent on their husbands. For these women, the Australian government provides a means-tested pension — often their only financial support. Whilst the husband is alive it is paid to him to provide health care services for both of them.

Cultural differences may also inhibit the access of non English speaking background women to health care services, and more particularly culturally appropriate services. In the case of migrant women, their second language, English, is often affected by language regression with age. In some cultures health care is mediated through the male partner, if he has not already died.

There may be a shortage of treatment services for women, as in the case of rural women. The South Australian Health Commission study (1990) of breast cancer showed that women living in rural areas who are aged 70 or over are more likely to die of breast cancer than their city counterparts with the same stage of disease. Travelling distance from specialised treatment was deemed to be an important factor in the outcome of this disease.

Physical access to health services is also a problem for urban elderly women. In the Women's Health Policy Review Committee Report of New South Wales (1985) reforms to the ambulance service, limiting the use of ambulances for non-acute work, were cited as a major inhibitor of access. Departments of Health, Transport and Local Government have not as yet addressed this shortfall.

Where services are available they are not necessarily appropriate. The difficulty in addressing the burden of chronic illness which women carry is reflected in the prescription and use of medications by older women. The Australian Consumers Association (1988) found in a survey of older consumers that there was an average of 4.76 medications per subject. Whilst the most common medications taken by older women are for the treatment of cardiovascular and respiratory illness, attention has focused on the potentially addictive medications prescribed to them, that is tranquillisers and hypnotics (see chapter ten).

STRATEGIES FOR OLDER WOMEN

Older women are clear about what they want from their health care systems. The Australian Council on the Ageing (ACOTA) believes that the current cohort of older women require strategies to be directed through doctors, as these women consider doctors as figures of high authority. ACOTA suggests that this strategy should not remain fixed and that older women over the next twenty years may require different strategies.

In 1989, Saltman, Webster and Therin identified three strategies integral to the health of older women, on the basis of interviews with older women in a non-health care environment. Subjects were asked to define their health in a non-medical way. What became clear from these exploratory interviews is that older women know what makes them feel healthy. The strategies are as follows:

Activities and interests. Older women were concerned about health and how to keep it centred on maintaining an active, mobile lifestyle. The following activities were mentioned in descending order of frequency: sleeping, swimming, walking, gardening, housework and showering.

Whilst physical activities were of primary importance, the notion of interests reflected activities not wholly related to or limited by their physical capacities. Interests included: a balanced diet, music, alcohol, good weather, knitting, reading, listening to the radio and watching television.

It is clear that older women can identify health related activities which are more specific to their age group than those popularised in media programs.

Contacts and communication. Integral to any active lifestyle was a sense of belonging to a community. Specified company included: family, especially grandchildren, who 'kept them young', friends and pets. The interviewees reflected Kuhn's notions of a coalition of ageing and Mauss's analogy of a gift relationship within families, in a practical way.

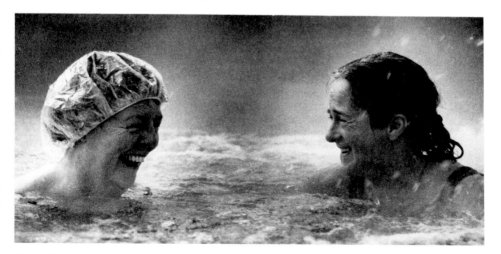

Physical activities are important to older women as are relationships with friends and family

Communication was the method by which the women maintained their associations with their contacts. Conversation and sharing problems was very important in the maintenance of health.

Independence and mental health. Less frequently cited was the concept of independence as a symptom of health. Comments such as 'having my own routine', 'looking after myself', 'staying out of nursing homes' and 'control over my own life' reflected the value the women placed on the level of independence they maintained.

The subjects held strongly negative attitudes towards nursing homes. Braun and Rose (1987) found in their study of outcomes for older patients in the areas of activities of daily living, mobility, morbidity, well-being, and cost that there were significantly better outcomes within an at home group compared with a nursing home group.

A wide range of ideas were mentioned in relation to mental health. They included:

- validation by society;
- feeling calm;
- invigorated, really great, clear headed, clean, fresh and proud of oneself;
- having a good mental outlook and a mind at rest; and
- believing health equals life.

The interviewees placed great importance on the pathways of their lives, memories were important and most of all a sense of satisfaction and achievement.

The role of the health care provider was to offer reassurance and information. These views are accurately summed up by older women as follows:

Because of bodily changes we may not be as fit as we used to be but we do not want to be treated as imbeciles. After all, we do have minds and for most of us they still work very well (Anderson and Luxford).

CASE STUDY

Edith is 76 years old, and still lives on the farm she and her husband, Bob, bought 50 years ago. Bob died two years ago, but she has continued to live in her own home, although now it really is the home of her son, who manages the property. He and his wife and three children moved into the homestead from their cottage when her husband died. It wasn't that she couldn't exactly manage for herself, it was more that the house was big, with a better garden for the children, and the farm office was already set up there. However, sometimes recently, she has felt very lonely in her own home. It doesn't seem to be hers any more, and her grandchildren are hard on the furniture she used to care for so painstakingly. They knocked over one of her favourite plants in the garden a few weeks ago — a shrub that she had nurtured carefully for years. What was troubling was that her daughter-in-law, Ann, didn't seem to realise the significance of that shrub, and didn't really reprimand the children for damaging it. The children are very tiring and she doesn't think Mike and Ann discipline them quite enough.

Last week Edith got out of bed at 5 o'clock in the morning to go to the toilet. As she got out of bed her leg seemed to give way beneath her, and she soon realised that her left hip was hurting dreadfully — she could not move. Ann ran into the room, having been woken by the sound of her fall. It was clear that Edith had hurt her leg badly, and so they made her comfortable on the floor, and waited till their family doctor came. He arranged for her admission to the local hospital, when an Xray confirmed a fracture of the neck of her femur. After a few days in hospital Edith seemed to be making good progress, although she was finding it difficult to be in bed, when she was used to being very active.

Then last weekend things changed. Edith became more and more restless and confused. Her mental state deteriorated quickly, and she did not even recognise her own grandchildren when they visited, and began to think Mike was her late husband. Mike was very worried about how they would cope if his mother returned home, as apparently she was neither physically nor mentally able to be an active member of the family. The worst part was that when they visited her, Edith just asked constantly to be taken out of hospital.

The only solution seemed to be to give her some of the sedative pills that the young hospital doctor said were available to help elderly people like Edith, and see if she could be taken in to the nursing home for the elderly in the town where the hospital was. Mike and Ann were finding it a strain to visit her in the hospital and keep the farm and the family going. Yet in the nursing home they would not be able to visit much, although Edith has some friends in town — but not too many.

While discussing the situation after dinner tonight, Ann decided to call one of her old school friends who was a physiotherapist with an assessment and rehabilitation service for the elderly in a town a few hundred kilometres away.

They spoke for a while, but Ann was even more mixed up when she came off the phone. Her friend was horrified to hear that the young doctor had mentioned a rest home because of Edith's confusion. This was not an uncommon occurrence in older people associated with an acute illness, she said, and only after very careful assessment of all aspects of Edith's life should a decision like that be made. She suggested they contact their family doctor, and clarify the plan of management with him.

The whole situation was frustrating and very worrying ....

REFERENCES

Anderson J. & Luxford Y. (1988). The coming out of older women, in *Community development in health project*, Community Development in Health 1988, Preston/Northcote District Health Council.

Anderson, W.F. (1981). Is health education for the middle-aged and elderly a waste of time? *Family and community health*, 3, 1–10.

Australian Bureau of Statistics (1982). *Australian health survey 1977–78*, AGPS, Canberra.

Australian Consumers Association and Combined Pensioners Association (1988). *Too much of a good thing: older consumers and their medications*, February, Australian Consumers Association, Sydney.

Australian Institute of Health (1988). *Australia's health*, First biennial report of the Australian Institute of Health, AGPS, Canberra.

Braithwaite, V. (1986). The burden of home care: how is it shared? in *Supplement to Community health studies*, X, 3.

Braun, K.L. & Rose, C.L. (1987). Geriatric patient outcomes and costs in three settings: nursing home, foster family, own home, *Journal of the American geriatric society*, 35, 387–97.

Hicks, N. (1986). Social policy, research on aging and aged care in Australia, In *Supplement to community health studies*, pp 1–86.

Johnson, M. (1975). Old age and the gift relationship, *New society*, March 13th.

Kinnear, D. & Graycar, A. (1982). Family care of elderly people: Australian perspectives, *Social Welfare Research Centre reports and proceedings*, 23, Social Welfare Research Centre, University of New South Wales.

Kuhn, M. (1977). *On aging*, Westminster Press, USA.

Lesnoff-Caravaglia, G. & Klys, M.L. (1987). An alternative paradigm for the study of aging, Letters to the editor, *JAGS*, 35, 366–7.

Mauss, M. (1954). *The gift*, The Free Press, London.

McPherson-Turner, C. (1980). Education for aging, *Journal of the school of health*, 314–6.

Philips, T. (1984). Cheaper is always less costly, In A. Graycar (ed.) *Accommodation after retirement, Social Welfare Research Centre reports and proceedings*, 41, Social Welfare Research Centre, University of New South Wales.

Rural women suffer (1990). *Australian doctor*, 16th February, p 25.

Saltman, D.C., Webster, I.W. & Therin, G.A. (1989). Older persons' definitions of good health: implications for general practitioners, *The medical journal of Australia*, 150, 426–8.

Webster, I.W. (1980). *Old age*, School of community medicine, University of New South Wales, Kensington.

Women's Health Policy Review Committee (1985). *Women's health services in New South Wales: final report*, Department of Health, New South Wales.

Index

Numbers in italics refer to tables and figures

3 4 5 6 7 8 9
B C D E F G H I J